I0074644

# CRAZY MEDICAL STORIES

## VOLUME 2

## DR. ERIN SMITH

FREE REIGN
Publishing

Copyright © 2024 by Erin Smith, M.D.
Published by Free Reign Publishing

This book or any portion thereof may not be reproduced or used in any
manner whatsoever without the express written permission of the
publisher except for the use of brief quotations in a book review. All
rights reserved.

ISBN 13: 979-8-89234-070-0

Free Reign Publishing, LLC
San Diego, CA

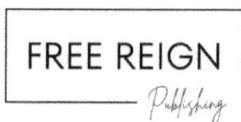

# CONTENTS

# INTRODUCTION

Welcome to the enthralling pages of *Crazy Medical Stories*, a captivating anthology series meticulously curated by the esteemed Dr. Erin Smith. With over two decades of extensive experience in the medical field, Dr. Smith has witnessed the extraordinary, the bewildering, and the downright inexplicable. In this remarkable collection, she brings together a series of incredible stories that promise to astonish, amuse, and perhaps even baffle readers.

*Crazy Medical Stories* is not just a compilation of medical anomalies; it is a testament to the unpredictability of human health, the complexity of our bodies, and the unyielding spirit of those who devote their lives to caring for others. Dr. Smith's journey through the labyrinth of medicine has equipped her with a treasure trove of experiences, each story serving as a unique thread in the rich tapestry of her career.

As you delve into these pages, you will find tales of resilience and resourcefulness, bizarre medical mysteries, and instances of serendipity that defy explanation. Dr. Smith's narrative is imbued with a sense of wonder and respect for the field of medicine, coupled with an unwavering commitment to her patients. Her storytelling prowess brings each case to life, allowing readers to step into her shoes and experience the whirlwind of emotions that accompany each medical adventure.

Beyond the captivating stories, this anthology serves as a reflection on the art of medicine itself. It highlights the importance of empathy, intuition, and the relentless pursuit of knowledge. Dr. Smith's anecdotes underscore the fact that, in medicine, sometimes the journey to a diagnosis is just as fascinating as the diagnosis itself.

So, buckle up and prepare for a roller coaster ride through the world of medicine like you've never experienced before. Whether you are a medical professional, a student of medicine, or simply a curious reader with a penchant for the extraordinary, *Crazy Medical Stories* promises to be a journey filled with awe, laughter, and a renewed appreciation for the unexpected twists and turns of life. Welcome to the world through the eyes of Dr. Erin Smith—a world where the line between the possible and the improbable is wonderfully blurred.

# CHAPTER ONE

## L1 SYNDROME

I REMEMBER THE DAY CLEARLY, one of those unusually warm autumn afternoons when the sun seems reluctant to leave the sky. The patient was referred to me, a seemingly ordinary individual who had begun to experience a series of inexplicable symptoms. The signs were subtle at first, a slight weakness in the legs, a clumsiness that had never been present before. But as the weeks passed, the symptoms progressed with alarming speed. The patient's movements grew more labored, and the once simple act of walking became a strenuous task.

The initial tests showed nothing conclusive, and the early misdiagnoses ranged from multiple sclerosis to peripheral neuropathy. It wasn't until the patient underwent a thorough neurological examination that the possibility of L1 Syndrome emerged. The syndrome, a rare genetic disorder, affects the nervous system and can lead to a host of complications, including spasticity, intellectual disability, and varying degrees of paralysis.

The patient's condition had begun to deteriorate at a pace that suggested a more aggressive form of the disease. When I first broached the topic of genetic testing, there was a glimmer of hope in their eyes—a hope that perhaps there would be an answer, something tangible to fight against. The test results confirmed our suspicions: the patient had L1 Syndrome, a mutation in the L1CAM gene. The diagnosis was a double-edged sword; it provided an answer but also outlined a grim prognosis.

The treatment plan was comprehensive but not curative. The primary goal was to manage symptoms and improve the quality of life as much as possible. Physical therapy was initiated immediately to address the increasing spasticity and maintain mobility for as long as possible. The patient showed remarkable determination during these sessions, pushing through the pain and frustration that accompanied each exercise. Despite the physical limitations, the spirit within remained undaunted.

Medication was another cornerstone of the treatment. Antispasmodics were prescribed to reduce muscle stiffness, while anticonvulsants were introduced to manage the seizures that had begun to manifest. The patient responded reasonably well to the medications, but the side effects were significant. There were days when the fatigue from the drugs seemed almost as debilitating as the symptoms they were meant to control.

As the disease progressed, the patient required more intensive care. A multidisciplinary approach was adopted, involving neurologists, physiotherapists, occupational therapists, and speech therapists. Each specialist contributed to creating a tailored plan to address the unique challenges posed by L1 Syndrome. Adaptive equipment was introduced to aid mobility, and home modifications were made to ensure safety and accessibility.

The patient's cognitive abilities also began to decline, a heart-wrenching development that added another layer of complexity to the treatment. Memory lapses became more frequent, and simple tasks that were once performed with ease now required detailed instructions. The occupational therapist worked tirelessly to develop strategies to maintain cognitive function and independence. Memory aids, structured routines, and engaging activities were all part of the daily regimen.

Throughout the treatment, regular monitoring was crucial. MRI scans were conducted periodically to assess any changes in the brain's structure, and blood tests were done to ensure the medications were not causing harm to other organs. The patient's health was a delicate balance, and even the slightest misstep could lead to severe consequences.

Despite the rigorous treatment plan, the disease continued its relentless march. The patient's mobility declined further, and soon a wheelchair became a necessity. The transition was challenging, both physically and emotionally. The once vibrant individual who had walked into my office months ago was now grappling with a body that seemed to betray them at every turn. Yet, through it all, there remained an indomitable strength, a fierce determination to make the most of each day.

The patient's family played an integral role in the treatment process. Their support was unwavering, and their presence provided a source of comfort and motivation. They attended therapy sessions, learned how to assist with exercises, and adapted their lives to accommodate the new normal. The bond between the patient and their family was palpable, a testament to the power of love and solidarity in the face of adversity.

As the disease entered its final stages, the focus of treatment shifted to palliative care. The goal was no longer to fight the inevitable but to ensure that the patient's remaining days were as comfortable and meaningful as possible. Pain management became a priority, with careful adjustments to medication to balance efficacy and side effects. The patient was enrolled in a hospice program, where they received compassionate care from a team of dedicated professionals.

Throughout this journey, there were moments of profound beauty and grace. The patient's resilience was inspiring, their spirit unbroken even as their body weakened. They found joy in small pleasures—listening to their favorite music, spending time with loved ones, and reminiscing about happier times. These moments were a poignant reminder of the human capacity to find light even in the darkest of times.

As a doctor, witnessing the patient's journey was both a privilege and a profound lesson in the fragility and strength of the human condition. The medical interventions, while necessary, were only one aspect of the care provided. Equally important were the emotional and psychological support, the reassurance, and the moments of shared humanity that transcended the clinical environment.

The patient's decline was gradual yet inevitable. The days grew shorter, the nights longer, filled with a quiet anticipation of the end. When the time finally came, it was peaceful. Surrounded by family, the patient passed away with a sense of dignity and grace. Their journey, though marked by suffering, was also a testament to the human spirit's ability to endure and find meaning even in the face of insurmountable odds.

In reflecting on the patient's journey, I was reminded of the profound impact that a single life can have. Despite the challenges posed by L1 Syndrome, the patient's courage and determination left an indelible mark on everyone who had the privilege of knowing them. The medical journey from diagnosis to treatment, and ultimately to the end of life, was a stark reminder of the limits of medicine and the boundless capacity of the human spirit to endure and inspire.

# CHAPTER TWO

## CONGENITAL ROD DISEASE

THE DAY BEGAN like any other in the clinic, a quiet morning punctuated by the sound of pages turning and the hum of the fluorescent lights above. As I flipped through the latest medical journal, my mind half-occupied by the article on emerging gene therapies, the nurse knocked lightly on my door. She handed me the patient file with a grave look that hinted at something more than the usual cases of seasonal flu or minor injuries.

The patient had been referred to us after a routine eye exam had raised some serious concerns. Born with Congenital Rod Disease, a rare genetic disorder that affects the photoreceptor cells in the retina, the patient had lived with deteriorating vision since childhood. Congenital Rod Disease, as I well knew, leads to night blindness and tunnel vision, and in some cases, can result in complete loss of sight.

As I read through the file, the patient's history unfolded before me. From an early age, it was clear that there was something different about their vision. In dim light, the patient stumbled frequently and had difficulty recognizing faces or navigating unfamiliar environments. As the years progressed, the challenges multiplied, and the once bright and lively child became increasingly withdrawn, struggling to keep up with their peers in school and everyday activities.

When the patient entered my office, I noted the tentative steps and the way their eyes seemed to scan the room, searching for a familiar anchor. I introduced myself and gestured for them to take a seat. The patient's anxiety was palpable, a thin thread woven through their careful movements and the tight grip on the edge of the chair.

I began with a thorough examination, assessing the patient's visual acuity, field of vision, and response to different levels of light. As expected, the tests confirmed significant impairment. The patient's night vision was virtually nonexistent, and the peripheral vision was severely restricted. The rods, which are responsible for low-light vision, had degenerated to the point where only the central field remained somewhat functional.

With the initial examination complete, I explained the need for further tests. We scheduled an electroretinography (ERG) to measure the electrical responses of the retina's photoreceptors. This test would give us a clearer picture of the extent of rod dysfunction and help us understand the progression of the disease. The patient listened quietly, nodding at intervals, their expression a mix of resignation and hope.

The ERG results were as anticipated, revealing a significant reduction in rod function. This confirmed the diagnosis of Congenital Rod Disease. While the condition was irreversible, there were treatment options available to slow the progression and potentially improve the patient's quality of life. I discussed these options in detail, outlining the pros and cons of each approach.

The primary treatment involved the use of vitamin A supplements, which had shown some promise in slowing the degeneration of the photoreceptors. Additionally, we considered the use of specialized glasses that could enhance the patient's remaining vision by filtering certain wavelengths of light. These glasses would not restore vision but could help the patient navigate more easily in low-light conditions.

Gene therapy, a burgeoning field at the time, also offered a glimmer of hope. Though still in experimental stages, early trials had shown that introducing healthy copies of the defective gene into the retina could potentially halt or even reverse some of the damage. I explained that this option was not without risks and would require careful consideration and monitoring.

The patient opted to start with the less invasive treatments, beginning a regimen of vitamin A supplements and acquiring a pair of the specialized glasses. Over the following months, we monitored their progress closely. The supplements appeared to slow the rate of degeneration, and the glasses provided some improvement in daily activities. The patient reported fewer difficulties in navigating their home and felt more confident venturing out in the evenings.

Despite these small victories, the disease continued its relentless march. The patient's central vision, once a reliable stronghold, began to falter. Reading became a struggle, even with magnification, and the patient increasingly relied on auditory cues and touch to compensate for the loss. The psychological toll was evident, as the patient grappled with the reality of their condition and the limitations it imposed.

After a year of conventional treatments, the patient expressed a desire to explore the possibility of gene therapy. The decision was not made lightly, as the risks and uncertainties were significant. We proceeded with a battery of pre-therapy evaluations to ensure the patient was a suitable candidate. These tests included genetic sequencing to confirm the specific mutation responsible for the disease, as well as a comprehensive assessment of the patient's overall health.

The results were encouraging, and the patient was deemed eligible for the experimental procedure. The therapy involved injecting a viral vector carrying the healthy gene directly into the retina. This delicate process required precision and expertise, and the patient would need to remain under close observation for several weeks post-procedure to monitor for adverse reactions and complications.

The day of the procedure arrived, and the patient was prepped for surgery. As I stood by, overseeing the process, I marveled at the strides medical science had made in such a short time. The surgeon skillfully administered the injection, and we all held our breath, hoping for the best.

The initial recovery period was uneventful, with no immediate complications. Over the next few weeks, we monitored the patient's progress with bated breath. Early signs were promising; there was no rejection or inflammation, and the patient reported subtle improvements in their vision. Shadows and shapes that had once been indistinguishable began to take form, and the patient's confidence grew with each passing day.

As the months wore on, the improvements became more pronounced. The patient's night vision, while not fully restored, was markedly better. They could navigate dimly lit environments with relative ease, and their peripheral vision, though still limited, showed signs of improvement. The patient's quality of life improved significantly, and they began to reclaim activities and hobbies that had once seemed out of reach.

The journey, however, was far from smooth. There were setbacks and moments of despair when progress seemed to stall or even regress. Each time, the patient met these challenges with a determination that was truly remarkable. The support of family and friends played a crucial role, providing a network of encouragement and assistance that bolstered the patient's spirits.

After a year of post-therapy monitoring, it became clear that the gene therapy had made a significant impact. While the patient's vision was not perfect, it was vastly improved compared to the pre-therapy state. The once inevitable march towards blindness had been halted, and the patient was granted a reprieve, a chance to experience life with a clarity they had long thought lost.

Reflecting on the journey, I couldn't help but feel a deep sense of fulfillment. The patient's story was a testament to the power of medical science and the indomitable human spirit. It reminded me why I had chosen this profession, to witness and contribute to the profound moments of healing and hope.

As the patient left my office for the final follow-up appointment, their steps were more assured, their gaze more focused. The path ahead was still fraught with challenges, but they faced it with a renewed sense of purpose and courage. Their story, a beacon of hope and perseverance, would stay with me always, a reminder of the miracles that can happen when science and the human spirit come together in pursuit of a common goal.

# CHAPTER THREE

## ROSENFELD-KLOEPFER SYNDROME

THE PATIENT WAS REFERRED to my care after a series of baffling symptoms had left their general practitioner at a loss. Upon their arrival, the patient exhibited a striking combination of neurological and dermatological manifestations, symptoms so rare and severe that I suspected Rosenfeld-Kloepfer syndrome almost immediately. The patient's medical history revealed an insidious onset of symptoms, beginning with mild sensory disturbances and gradually progressing to severe neurological deficits and widespread skin abnormalities.

The patient's hands trembled as they explained their journey through a myriad of tests and consultations, each yielding inconclusive results. It was the gradual progression from mild to severe that caught my attention. Their skin, once unremarkable, now bore the hallmark lesions and plaques associated with Rosenfeld-Kloepfer syndrome. The neurological symptoms—muscle weakness, coordination problems, and cognitive decline—painted a clear picture of a degenerative process that was relentless and unforgiving.

Upon conducting a thorough examination, I noted the patient's ataxia, a distinct lack of coordination that made simple tasks arduous. Their gait was unsteady, and their speech, once fluid, had become slurred and difficult to understand. The skin lesions were numerous, scattered across their body in a seemingly haphazard pattern, each one a testament to the disease's destructive nature. The patient's eyes, though bright with intelligence, betrayed an underlying fear and uncertainty, a fear that I shared but could not express.

The diagnostic process was rigorous. I ordered a battery of tests, including an MRI to assess the extent of neurological damage, and a biopsy of the skin lesions to confirm the diagnosis. The MRI results were telling—marked atrophy in the cerebellum and widespread demyelination indicated significant neurological compromise. The biopsy results, too, were conclusive, revealing the characteristic changes in skin tissue associated with the syndrome.

Breaking the news to the patient was a task I approached with a heavy heart. Despite my years of experience, delivering a diagnosis of Rosenfeld-Kloepfer syndrome was never easy. I explained the nature of the disease, its progression, and the limited treatment options available. The patient's face remained stoic, absorbing each word with a silent resignation that spoke volumes. It was clear they had suspected something severe but had hoped for a less dire reality.

Treatment for Rosenfeld-Kloepfer syndrome is largely symptomatic, as there is no cure. Our goal was to manage the symptoms and improve the patient's quality of life as much as possible. The multidisciplinary approach involved neurologists, dermatologists, physical therapists, and occupational therapists. Each specialist played a crucial role in addressing the various facets of the disease.

The neurological symptoms required immediate attention. We initiated a regimen of medications aimed at slowing the progression of the neurological decline. Immunosuppressive drugs were introduced to modulate the immune response, which was believed to play a role in the disease's progression. Physical therapy was essential to maintain as much motor function as possible. The patient's sessions were intensive, focusing on balance, coordination, and muscle strength. Despite the rigorous nature of these sessions, the patient attended each one with a determination that was both admirable and heart-breaking.

The dermatological aspect of the disease was equally challenging. The skin lesions were treated with a combination of topical corticosteroids and systemic medications to reduce inflammation and slow the progression of the lesions. Regular visits to the dermatologist became a part of the patient's routine, each session a battle against the relentless advancement of the disease.

As weeks turned into months, the patient's condition fluctuated. There were days when the treatments seemed to hold the disease at bay, allowing moments of reprieve from the relentless symptoms. On other days, the disease's progression seemed unstoppable, each new symptom a stark reminder of the battle being fought. The patient's cognitive functions deteriorated slowly but noticeably. Simple tasks became increasingly difficult, and conversations, once engaging and thoughtful, grew fragmented and confused.

Despite these challenges, the patient's spirit remained remarkably steadfast. They adhered to the treatment regimen with an unwavering commitment, attending every appointment and following every recommendation. Their family, too, played an instrumental role, providing support and care that was both tender and unyielding. It was clear that the patient's journey was not one they walked alone, but one shared with loved ones who bore the weight of the disease alongside them.

The passage of time brought with it an inevitable decline. The patient's neurological symptoms worsened, and the physical therapy sessions, once a means of maintaining function, became exercises in maintaining dignity and comfort. The ataxia progressed to the point where walking unaided was no longer possible, and the patient required assistance with even the most basic of tasks. The skin lesions, despite aggressive treatment, continued to spread and worsen, causing pain and discomfort that was managed with an ever-increasing array of medications.

Throughout this time, my role was one of both clinician and confidant. I monitored the patient's physical and cognitive status, adjusted treatments as necessary, and provided support and guidance to both the patient and their family. Each visit was a reminder of the disease's relentless nature, yet also a testament to the human capacity for endurance in the face of overwhelming odds.

As the disease progressed, palliative care became an increasingly important aspect of the treatment plan. The focus shifted from attempting to slow the disease to ensuring the patient's comfort and quality of life. Pain management became a priority, as did addressing the emotional and psychological toll of the disease. The patient's world grew smaller as their mobility and cognitive functions declined, yet their interactions with their loved ones remained a source of comfort and connection.

In the final stages of the disease, the patient's condition deteriorated rapidly. Neurological decline left them bedridden, and communication became difficult. The skin lesions, now widespread and painful, were managed with a combination of pain relief and topical treatments aimed at minimizing discomfort. The patient's family remained a constant presence, their support and care unwavering even as the end drew near.

The patient passed away surrounded by loved ones, their final moments a testament to the strength and dedication of those who had supported them throughout their journey. The experience left an indelible mark on all involved, a poignant reminder of the fragility of life and the profound impact of illness.

# CHAPTER FOUR

## MEYENBURG-ALTHERR-UEHLINGER SYNDROME

AS A PHYSICIAN SPECIALIZING in rare diseases, I encountered numerous patients with uncommon syndromes. Each case presented unique challenges, but none were quite as enigmatic as the patient diagnosed with Meyenburg-Altherr-Uehlinger syndrome. This account details the journey from diagnosis through treatment, revealing the struggles faced by the patient and the medical team's relentless efforts to alleviate the symptoms of this rare condition.

The patient, a middle-aged individual, arrived at my clinic with a complex array of symptoms. They presented with severe abdominal pain, unexplained weight loss, and chronic fatigue. Initial examinations and routine tests revealed little. However, the persistence of symptoms suggested something more profound. Suspecting an underlying liver disorder, I ordered a comprehensive liver panel and an abdominal ultrasound. The results showed mildly elevated liver enzymes and a few irregularities, but nothing definitive.

Not satisfied with these inconclusive findings, I decided to proceed with more advanced imaging studies. A contrast-enhanced CT scan was performed, revealing multiple cystic lesions scattered throughout the liver. These findings raised my suspicion of polycystic liver disease, but the patient's symptoms and presentation did not entirely match this diagnosis. A more nuanced investigation was required.

A liver biopsy was the next step. The procedure, though invasive, was necessary to gain a clearer understanding of the hepatic abnormalities. The biopsy samples were sent for histopathological examination. Days of anxious waiting followed, both for me and the patient, as we anticipated the results that would hopefully shed light on the perplexing condition.

The biopsy report arrived, bearing the hallmark findings of Meyenburg-Altherr-Uehlinger syndrome: multiple bile duct hamartomas. These benign lesions, though typically asymptomatic, had proliferated extensively in the patient's liver, leading to the array of debilitating symptoms. The diagnosis was confirmed, but this was just the beginning of our arduous journey.

Meyenburg-Altherr-Uehlinger syndrome, a rare congenital condition, often goes unnoticed due to its typically silent nature. However, in this case, the extensive growth of bile duct hamartomas had caused significant disruption. The patient's liver function was compromised, and the cystic lesions were exerting pressure on surrounding tissues, exacerbating the symptoms. Understanding the rarity and the complex pathophysiology of this syndrome, I knew that treatment options were limited and challenging.

Our primary goal was to alleviate the patient's symptoms and improve their quality of life. Surgical intervention was deemed too risky due to the extensive nature of the lesions and the potential for complications. Instead, we opted for a conservative approach focusing on symptom management and supportive care. A multidisciplinary team, including hepatologists, gastroenterologists, and pain management specialists, was assembled to devise a comprehensive treatment plan.

The initial phase of treatment involved managing the patient's pain, which was the most debilitating symptom. A regimen of analgesics and antispasmodic medications was prescribed to provide relief. Additionally, the patient was placed on a specialized diet to mitigate gastrointestinal symptoms and prevent further weight loss. Nutritional support, including high-calorie supplements and vitamins, was essential to bolster their weakened state.

Given the compromised liver function, monitoring and managing potential complications became a priority. Regular liver function tests and imaging studies were scheduled to track the progression of the lesions and any impact on liver health. The patient was also started on ursodeoxycholic acid, a bile acid derivative, in an attempt to improve bile flow and reduce hepatic stress.

Despite our efforts, the patient's condition remained precarious. The pain management strategy provided some relief, but the chronic fatigue and weight loss persisted. Over time, the patient developed symptoms of cholestasis, including jaundice and pruritus, indicating further deterioration of liver function. This necessitated the introduction of additional medications to manage these complications and provide symptomatic relief.

In parallel with medical treatment, the patient received psychological support. The chronic nature of the illness and the physical limitations it imposed took a toll on their mental health. Regular counseling sessions were arranged to help them cope with the emotional burden of living with a chronic, debilitating condition.

Months passed with little improvement. The patient's condition fluctuated, showing brief periods of stabilization followed by sudden declines. The relentless progression of the syndrome challenged our medical expertise and tested the patient's fortitude. Every slight improvement was a beacon of hope, only to be dimmed by the recurrent setbacks.

During one particularly severe episode, the patient was hospitalized with acute liver failure. The cystic lesions had grown, obstructing bile flow and leading to a buildup of toxins in the bloodstream. Intensive care was required to stabilize the patient, involving intravenous fluids, electrolytes, and medications to support liver function. The situation was dire, and the prognosis was uncertain.

The multidisciplinary team convened once again to reassess the treatment strategy. It became clear that conventional approaches were insufficient. We explored experimental treatments and clinical trials, seeking any potential avenues that could offer relief or at least slow the progression of the syndrome. However, the rarity of Meyenburg-Altherr-Uehlinger syndrome meant that research was limited, and viable options were few.

After weeks of intensive treatment, the patient's condition began to stabilize. Though still critically ill, the immediate threat of liver failure was averted. This respite, albeit temporary, provided an opportunity to reassess and fine-tune the ongoing treatment regimen. We intensified the supportive care measures, focusing on maintaining liver function and preventing further complications.

Over the following months, the patient's condition remained fragile. Regular monitoring and adjustments to the treatment plan became routine. Each day was a battle to balance symptom management and preserve liver function. The patient's strength and determination in the face of such adversity were remarkable, even as their body continued to betray them.

As time passed, the inevitable progression of the syndrome became more apparent. Despite our best efforts, the cystic lesions continued to grow, and liver function declined steadily. The patient's health deteriorated, and they became increasingly debilitated. The weight loss and chronic fatigue worsened, leaving them bedridden and dependent on constant care.

In the final stages of the disease, our focus shifted to palliative care. Ensuring the patient's comfort and dignity became our primary concern. Pain management was intensified, and additional measures were taken to address the jaundice and pruritus. The psychological support continued, providing solace during this profoundly challenging time.

Ultimately, despite all interventions, the patient succumbed to the syndrome. The complexity and relentless progression of Meyenburg-Altherr-Uehlinger syndrome had outpaced our medical capabilities. The patient's journey was a testament to the limits of modern medicine in the face of rare and intractable diseases.

The loss was profound, not only for the patient's family and loved ones but also for the medical team that had fought tirelessly to provide care. This case left an indelible mark on all of us, a stark reminder of the challenges inherent in treating rare diseases and the courage required to face them.

Each patient's journey with a rare syndrome like Meyenburg-Altherr-Uehlinger is unique, marked by both triumphs and tribulations. This particular case, with its complex diagnosis and arduous treatment path, highlighted the importance of perseverance and adaptability in medical practice. Though we could not alter the course of the disease, the efforts to alleviate suffering and maintain dignity until the end were a testament to the essence of compassionate care.

Through this experience, I gained a deeper understanding of the intricacies of rare diseases and the profound impact they have on patients and their families. The patient's struggle, though ultimately ending in loss, underscored the critical need for continued research and innovation in the field of rare diseases. It is through such relentless pursuit of knowledge that we hope to find better treatments and, perhaps one day, a cure for those affected by syndromes like Meyenburg-Altherr-Uehlinger.

# CHAPTER FIVE

## BROKEN HEART SYNDROME

AS A NURSE, I've encountered countless patients, each one with their unique story, but few have touched me as deeply as the patient with broken heart syndrome. This particular case stands out, not only for its medical intricacies but for the profound emotional impact it had on everyone involved, including myself.

It was a gray, rainy morning when the patient was brought in. The paramedics reported chest pain and shortness of breath. Initially, everyone in the emergency room suspected a heart attack. The patient's vitals were unstable, and the rapid assessment showed signs pointing towards a myocardial infarction. The cardiologist on call ordered an immediate EKG and blood tests. As I prepared the patient for these tests, I couldn't help but notice the haunted look in their eyes, as if a weight heavier than mere physical pain was bearing down upon them.

The EKG results came back surprisingly normal, which was puzzling given the symptoms. The blood tests revealed mildly elevated cardiac enzymes, but not to the extent typically seen in a heart attack. The cardiologist, suspecting something amiss, ordered an echocardiogram. As the ultrasound waves mapped out the heart's structure and function, a striking pattern emerged. The apex of the heart was not contracting properly, a phenomenon known as apical ballooning. The cardiologist diagnosed the patient with Takotsubo cardiomyopathy, commonly referred to as broken heart syndrome.

Takotsubo cardiomyopathy mimics a heart attack but is usually triggered by extreme emotional or physical stress. The patient had experienced a traumatic event shortly before the onset of symptoms, which likely precipitated this condition. The heart's left ventricle temporarily weakened, leading to its distinctive balloon-like shape. Despite the initial scare, the condition was generally considered reversible with appropriate treatment.

The first step in the patient's treatment was stabilization. They were placed on medications to manage pain and reduce the heart's workload. Beta-blockers were prescribed to slow the heart rate and lower blood pressure, while ACE inhibitors helped relax blood vessels and improve blood flow. Diuretics were also given to reduce fluid buildup and alleviate pressure on the heart. Throughout this process, I monitored the patient closely, administering medications and ensuring they were comfortable.

Despite the gravity of the situation, I remained hopeful. I had seen patients recover from broken heart syndrome before, and with the right care, there was every reason to believe this patient would too. Over the next few days, the patient remained in the intensive care unit, where they were closely monitored. I was there for every shift, watching over them, adjusting medications, and providing the necessary support. The patient was cooperative but noticeably withdrawn, a silent testament to the emotional burden that had triggered their condition.

In the following week, the patient's condition began to improve. Their vitals stabilized, and they started responding well to the medication. An echocardiogram showed slight improvement in the heart's function, which was encouraging. However, recovery from Takotsubo cardiomyopathy isn't solely a physical journey; the emotional aspect is equally critical. The patient needed to confront and process the underlying trauma that had caused their heart to break, quite literally.

A team of mental health professionals was brought in to assist with this aspect of recovery. Psychiatrists and psychologists worked together to provide therapy and counseling. The patient's sessions focused on coping mechanisms and strategies to deal with stress. The aim was to build emotional fortitude, ensuring the patient could handle future stresses without a repeat of such a severe physical manifestation. As a nurse, I was often present during these sessions, not actively participating, but offering silent support and ensuring the patient felt safe.

Despite the promising physical recovery, the patient's emotional healing was slow. They remained reserved, and there were days when the weight of their trauma seemed insurmountable. But there were also moments of progress, glimpses of light breaking through the clouds of despair. It was during these moments that I felt a deep sense of empathy and connection with the patient. Their struggle was palpable, and I wished I could do more than administer medications and adjust IV lines.

Over the next month, the patient continued to improve. Their heart function returned to near-normal levels, and the cardiologist expressed optimism about a full physical recovery. Yet, the emotional scars were still evident. The patient's journey through therapy was arduous, filled with ups and downs. Each small victory in therapy was hard-won, but significant. The patient started to open up more, sharing bits of their story, and slowly, the heavy burden they carried seemed to lighten.

One afternoon, as I was doing my rounds, I noticed a change in the patient. There was a subtle shift in their demeanor, a flicker of hope in their eyes that hadn't been there before. They were engaging more with the mental health team, actively participating in their own recovery. This change, however slight, was a pivotal moment. It marked the beginning of a new chapter in their healing process, one where they were not just a passive recipient of care but an active participant.

Weeks turned into months, and the patient's progress continued. Their heart function was now completely normal, and they were no longer on the intensive regimen of medications. The focus shifted entirely to their emotional well-being. The patient was discharged from the hospital but continued with outpatient therapy. They were given tools and resources to help them manage stress and cope with their trauma. Follow-up appointments with the cardiologist confirmed that the heart was healthy, a testament to the patient's remarkable recovery.

As a nurse, this case left an indelible mark on me. The patient's journey was a profound reminder of the intricate connection between the mind and body. Their broken heart was not just a metaphorical expression of grief but a real, physical condition that demanded both medical and emotional healing. Witnessing their transformation was both humbling and inspiring. It underscored the importance of holistic care, where healing encompasses not just the physical ailment but the emotional and psychological wounds as well.

The patient's story did not end with a neat conclusion or a tidy reflection. Life is seldom that straightforward. Instead, it was an ongoing journey of healing and rediscovery. They left the hospital stronger in many ways, having faced the depths of their trauma and emerged with a newfound strength. Their recovery was a testament to the power of human endurance and the remarkable ability of the heart – both literal and metaphorical – to heal and endure.

# CHAPTER SIX

## VALINE TRANSAMINASE DEFICIENCY

I HAD BEEN PRACTICING medicine for over two decades, encountering a myriad of diseases and disorders that tested the limits of my knowledge and skills. Yet, it was a case of Valine Transaminase Deficiency that left an indelible mark on my memory, challenging my medical acumen in ways I had never anticipated.

The patient was brought to my attention through a referral from a general practitioner who had noticed some troubling signs. Initially, the patient had presented with symptoms that were vague yet concerning: chronic fatigue, muscle weakness, and an overall sense of malaise that seemed to have no definitive cause. These symptoms had been persistent for several months, gradually worsening despite various attempts at treatment for more common ailments.

Upon the patient's arrival at my clinic, I conducted a thorough physical examination, taking meticulous notes on every aspect of their condition. The patient, a middle-aged individual, appeared visibly drained, with a pallor that suggested a possible metabolic or hematologic disorder. My initial blood tests revealed elevated levels of certain amino acids, particularly valine, which hinted at an underlying metabolic issue.

Suspecting a potential metabolic disorder, I ordered a series of more specific tests, including a plasma amino acid profile and enzyme assays. The results were telling. The patient's plasma amino acid profile showed markedly elevated levels of valine, leucine, and isoleucine. Further enzyme assays confirmed a deficiency in the enzyme branched-chain $\alpha$-keto acid dehydrogenase complex (BCKD), crucial for the catabolism of these amino acids. This enzyme deficiency is characteristic of Maple Syrup Urine Disease (MSUD), a rare genetic disorder. However, the patient's urine did not have the characteristic sweet odor typical of MSUD, leading me to consider other possibilities.

Delving deeper, I explored the less common metabolic disorders, focusing on those that might present with similar biochemical profiles but distinct clinical manifestations. My research brought me to Valine Transaminase Deficiency, an exceedingly rare condition

characterized by the body's inability to properly metabo-
lize valine due to a deficiency in the enzyme valine
transaminase. The rarity of this disorder meant that literature on it was sparse, with only a handful of docu-
mented cases worldwide.

With a working diagnosis of Valine Transaminase
Deficiency, I initiated a treatment plan aimed at
managing the patient's symptoms and preventing the
buildup of toxic metabolites. The cornerstone of the
treatment was a carefully controlled diet low in valine,
designed to reduce the intake of this amino acid and thus
minimize the production of toxic byproducts. Collabo-
rating with a dietitian specializing in metabolic disorders, we developed a tailored dietary plan for the
patient, meticulously calculating the permissible levels
of valine.

In addition to dietary management, I prescribed a
regimen of supplements to address potential deficiencies
and support overall metabolic function. This included a
combination of vitamins and cofactors known to play a
role in amino acid metabolism, such as vitamin B6 (pyri-
doxine) and thiamine. Regular monitoring of the
patient's plasma amino acid levels became a critical
component of the treatment plan, allowing us to adjust
the dietary intake as needed.

The patient adhered to the prescribed dietary

restrictions with commendable determination, despite the challenges posed by such a stringent regimen. Over the following weeks, there were some encouraging signs of improvement. The patient reported a gradual decrease in muscle weakness and fatigue, and their overall energy levels began to stabilize. These initial improvements, while modest, were a testament to the efficacy of the dietary management and the patient's unwavering commitment.

However, the nature of Valine Transaminase Deficiency meant that progress was slow and fraught with setbacks. Periodic episodes of metabolic decompensation occurred, often triggered by seemingly minor dietary indiscretions or intercurrent illnesses. These episodes were characterized by acute exacerbations of symptoms, including profound fatigue, muscle pain, and, occasionally, mild confusion. During these times, immediate medical intervention was necessary to prevent further deterioration. I would adjust the dietary plan, often reducing the intake of other branched-chain amino acids (leucine and isoleucine) to minimize the metabolic burden.

As the months passed, the patient's condition began to stabilize more consistently. Regular follow-ups showed a gradual normalization of plasma valine levels, and the patient's overall health improved incrementally. The stringent dietary restrictions and close medical supervision were proving effective, albeit challenging to maintain over the long term.

Throughout this period, the patient's determination was nothing short of inspiring. They meticulously followed the dietary plan, kept detailed food diaries, and attended every follow-up appointment with diligence. This unwavering commitment played a crucial role in managing the disorder and preventing severe metabolic crises.

Despite these efforts, the unpredictable nature of Valine Transaminase Deficiency meant that the threat of metabolic decompensation was always present. Periodic adjustments to the treatment plan were necessary, often requiring collaboration with specialists in metabolic disorders and genetic counseling. The patient's family also played a vital role, providing essential support and assistance in managing the complex dietary regimen.

One particularly challenging episode occurred approximately eighteen months into the treatment. The patient contracted a viral infection, which precipitated a severe metabolic crisis. The infection triggered an acute catabolic state, leading to a rapid increase in plasma valine levels and a corresponding exacerbation of symptoms. The patient was admitted to the hospital, where intensive medical management was necessary to stabilize their condition.

During this critical period, the patient received intravenous fluids, glucose, and electrolyte replacements to counteract the metabolic imbalance. Close monitoring of blood parameters allowed us to adjust the treatment dynamically, addressing each metabolic derangement as it arose. This acute episode was a stark reminder of the fragility of the patient's condition and the constant vigilance required to manage such a rare and complex disorder.

After several weeks of intensive care and meticulous management, the patient's condition stabilized once again. They were discharged from the hospital with a revised dietary plan and a renewed emphasis on monitoring and prevention. The recovery from this episode was slow but steady, and the patient's resilience was evident in their determined approach to regaining health and stability.

The journey with Valine Transaminase Deficiency was a continuous learning process for both the patient and myself. Each setback provided valuable insights into the management of the disorder, and each period of stability was a testament to the effectiveness of the treatment plan. The patient's unwavering commitment and the support of their family were integral to the success of the treatment, demonstrating the importance of a holistic approach to managing rare metabolic disorders.

As the years passed, the patient continued to navigate the challenges of Valine Transaminase Deficiency with remarkable perseverance. The stringent dietary restrictions became a way of life, and regular medical follow-ups ensured that any deviations were promptly addressed. The collaborative approach, involving dietitians, geneticists, and other specialists, provided a comprehensive support system that was crucial in managing the disorder.

Through this experience, I gained a profound appreciation for the complexities of rare metabolic disorders and the importance of individualized care. Each patient's journey is unique, shaped by their circumstances, their commitment, and the support they receive. Valine Transaminase Deficiency, with its rarity and complexity, underscored the need for ongoing research and awareness to improve diagnosis and treatment for future patients.

Reflecting on this case, I realized that the journey with the patient had been one of mutual growth and learning. The challenges we faced together and the progress we made were a testament to the power of dedicated medical care and the strength of the human spirit. The patient's journey was far from over, but the progress made and the lessons learned provided a solid foundation for continued management and improvement.

# CHAPTER SEVEN

## FACIOGENITAL DYSPLASIA

THE PATIENT WAS one of those rare cases that left an indelible mark on my career. It began one cold winter morning when they were wheeled into my examination room, shrouded in an aura of silent desperation. The face was unusually structured: the nasal bridge was depressed, the midface appeared sunken, and the jawline was undersized. Immediately, my clinical instincts were on high alert. These facial anomalies were not merely cosmetic concerns; they signaled something deeper, a congenital condition that might be more complex than what appeared on the surface.

I conducted a thorough physical examination. The patient's history was unremarkable aside from recurring infections and developmental delays during childhood. As I continued the examination, I noticed genital anomalies as well. The patient had ambiguous genitalia, a fact that had undoubtedly caused significant distress throughout their life. These combined findings pointed towards a rare genetic disorder, one that I had encountered only in textbooks and medical journals: faciogenital dysplasia, also known as Aarskog-Scott syndrome.

Faciogenital dysplasia is a disorder primarily affecting males, characterized by a constellation of features including distinctive facial morphology, skeletal abnormalities, and genital malformations. The pathophysiology is linked to mutations in the FGD1 gene located on the X chromosome, which disrupts normal cellular signaling pathways. Despite the known genetic basis, the condition manifests with a broad spectrum of severity, making each case unique.

The next step was to confirm the diagnosis through genetic testing. Blood samples were drawn and sent to the lab for sequencing of the FGD1 gene. The wait for the results felt interminable, not only for the patient but also for me. During this period, I gathered as much information as possible about their medical history, family background, and the challenges they had faced. Their medical history was riddled with frequent hospital visits for various infections and corrective surgeries that had provided only temporary relief.

When the genetic test results arrived, they

confirmed my suspicions. A mutation in the FGD1 gene was indeed present. With the diagnosis confirmed, the next challenge was devising a treatment plan. Faciogenital dysplasia is a lifelong condition with no cure, and management primarily focuses on symptomatic relief and improving the quality of life. I assembled a multidisciplinary team, including a geneticist, endocrinologist, urologist, and a psychologist, to address the multifaceted needs of the patient.

The initial focus was on the genital anomalies. The patient had undergone previous surgeries to correct hypospadias and cryptorchidism, but these had been only partially successful. The urologist suggested a more comprehensive reconstructive surgery to correct the remaining anomalies. This surgery was complex, involving delicate reconstruction to provide not only functional but also cosmetic improvement. The procedure took several hours, and the postoperative period was critical. The patient had to be monitored for infections and complications, a task that required meticulous care.

During the postoperative period, the patient's recovery was slow but steady. Pain management and infection control were our primary concerns. The patient was put on a regimen of antibiotics to prevent infections, and analgesics were administered to manage pain. Regular follow-ups were scheduled to monitor healing and ensure that the surgery was successful. The physical healing was one aspect, but addressing the psychological impact of their condition was equally important.

The psychologist worked closely with the patient, helping them navigate the emotional turmoil that had been a constant companion throughout their life. The sessions were intense and required a compassionate yet firm approach. They dealt with issues of self-esteem, social anxiety, and the trauma of repeated surgical interventions. It was a slow process, akin to peeling back layers of a deeply ingrained psychological wound, but progress was visible over time.

In parallel, the endocrinologist monitored the patient's hormonal levels. Faciogenital dysplasia often comes with endocrine abnormalities, such as delayed puberty or hormonal imbalances. Blood tests revealed that the patient had low levels of testosterone. Hormone replacement therapy (HRT) was initiated to address this deficiency. The endocrinologist carefully calibrated the dosage, aiming to mimic the body's natural hormonal rhythms. Regular blood tests were conducted to monitor the effectiveness of the therapy and adjust dosages as needed.

The facial anomalies required another set of interventions. Orthodontic treatment was necessary to correct dental misalignments caused by the abnormal jaw structure. Braces were fitted, and the patient had to endure the discomfort and inconvenience they brought. The orthodontist projected a treatment timeline of several years, during which regular adjustments would be necessary.

Surgical intervention was also planned to address the facial skeletal abnormalities. The maxillofacial surgeon proposed a series of osteotomies to reconstruct the midface and jaw. This surgery was perhaps the most daunting, involving high risks and a long recovery period. The patient was prepared for the procedure through extensive counseling and preoperative assessments. The surgery itself was a marathon, lasting over ten hours. The immediate postoperative period was fraught with complications. The patient experienced significant swelling, pain, and difficulty in breathing due to the extensive nature of the surgery. Intensive care support was critical during the initial days.

As the weeks passed, the swelling gradually subsided, and the new facial structure began to emerge. The transformation was profound, and although the patient's appearance would always carry the hallmark of their condition, the reconstruction provided a more balanced and symmetrical visage. Regular physiotherapy was needed to restore full functionality of the jaw and facial muscles. The patient diligently attended these sessions, despite the discomfort and slow progress.

Throughout this period, the patient's strength and determination were evident. They adhered to the rigorous treatment schedule, endured the physical pain, and participated actively in their recovery. This perseverance was a testament to their intrinsic fortitude, a quality that medical intervention alone could not provide. Their progress was a collaborative victory for the multidisciplinary team and a personal triumph for the patient.

Despite the significant improvements in physical appearance and functionality, the journey was far from over. The patient continued to face challenges, both medical and psychological. Regular monitoring and follow-ups became a permanent fixture in their life. The psychological support sessions transitioned from intensive therapy to periodic check-ins, ensuring that the patient had the resources to cope with any future challenges.

The final piece of the puzzle was social integration. The patient had spent a considerable portion of their life isolated due to the visible anomalies and the social stigma associated with them. Reintegrating into society required careful planning and support. Occupational therapy was introduced to help the patient develop skills for daily living and potential employment. Social skills training was also provided, focusing on building confidence and effective communication.

The patient's journey was marked by gradual, painstaking progress. Each small victory was celebrated, and setbacks were met with renewed determination. Over time, the physical scars faded, and the patient emerged with a renewed sense of self. The multidisciplinary approach had addressed the myriad aspects of their condition, providing a holistic treatment that went beyond mere physical correction.

As the years passed, the patient remained under regular medical supervision. The long-term management of faciogenital dysplasia required vigilance to prevent complications and address any new issues that arose. The patient's life had been irrevocably altered by their condition, but they had also found a path forward. Their story was one of relentless perseverance in the face of adversity, a narrative that highlighted the profound impact of comprehensive medical care.

The patient's case remains etched in my memory, not as a mere clinical challenge, but as a testament to the human spirit's capacity to endure and thrive despite overwhelming odds. The lessons learned from their treatment have informed my practice, underscoring the importance of a compassionate, multidisciplinary approach to complex congenital conditions. The journey was arduous, but it was also a powerful reminder of the difference that dedicated medical care can make in the lives of those affected by rare and challenging disorders.

# CHAPTER EIGHT

## CAROLI DISEASE

I HAD BEEN A PRACTICING physician for nearly twenty years when I first encountered Caroli Disease. It was an ordinary Wednesday when the patient was wheeled into my office. A middle-aged individual, appearing somewhat frail, who had been referred to me due to recurrent episodes of jaundice and severe abdominal pain. Their medical history was extensive, littered with episodes of cholangitis and repeated hospital admissions, which had been dismissed as simple gallstone disease by previous physicians.

The patient sat quietly as I reviewed their file, a thick bundle of papers chronicling years of misdiagnoses and ineffective treatments. I began my examination with a sense of unease, aware that something crucial had been overlooked. As I palpated their abdomen, the patient winced. I noted tenderness in the right upper quadrant, a telltale sign that something was amiss in the biliary system.

I ordered a series of imaging studies, including an ultrasound and an MRI cholangiopancreatography (MRCP). The ultrasound revealed dilated intrahepatic bile ducts, but it was the MRCP that provided the most critical insight. The images displayed a strikingly irregular pattern of bile duct dilatation, interspersed with normal segments. This characteristic finding pointed unmistakably towards Caroli Disease, a rare congenital disorder affecting the bile ducts.

Caroli Disease, as I explained to my colleagues later, is a condition where the bile ducts in the liver are abnormally widened, leading to the formation of cysts that can become infected. This not only results in recurrent episodes of cholangitis but also increases the risk of developing bile duct stones and, eventually, liver cirrhosis or cholangiocarcinoma. It was a diagnosis that carried significant implications for the patient's future.

Treatment for Caroli Disease is multifaceted and often complex. The first step in managing the patient's condition was addressing the acute cholangitis. I initiated broad-spectrum antibiotics to control the infection, and arranged for endoscopic retrograde cholangiopancreatography (ERCP) to drain the infected bile ducts.

The procedure was successful, and the patient's symptoms began to subside. However, I knew this was only a temporary solution.

Long-term management of Caroli Disease requires a combination of medical therapy and surgical intervention. I discussed the case with a hepatobiliary surgeon, and we decided that the patient would benefit from a partial hepatectomy. The idea was to resect the most severely affected segments of the liver, thus reducing the risk of recurrent cholangitis and other complications.

The patient underwent surgery a few weeks later. The operation was intricate, involving meticulous dissection around the dilated bile ducts to avoid injury to the remaining healthy liver tissue. The surgeon removed approximately one-third of the liver, including the sections with the most extensive cystic changes. Postoperative recovery was slow, marred by episodes of fever and mild liver dysfunction, but eventually, the patient began to stabilize.

In the following months, I monitored the patient closely. Their jaundice had resolved, and the abdominal pain was significantly reduced. We continued with periodic imaging studies to ensure there were no signs of recurrent disease. Despite the surgery, the patient remained at risk for complications such as cholangiocarcinoma, so we also implemented a regular screening program.

Unfortunately, six months post-surgery, the patient presented with new symptoms: weight loss, fatigue, and a dull ache in the right upper quadrant. A repeat MRCP showed a mass in the liver, suspicious for cholangiocarcinoma. The news was devastating. Caroli Disease, with its chronic inflammation and recurrent infections, had set the stage for this malignancy.

We embarked on a new treatment plan, this time focusing on the cancer. The patient underwent chemotherapy, a grueling regimen that took a toll on their already weakened body. Despite the aggressive treatment, the cancer progressed. It spread to the lymph nodes and eventually to the lungs.

As a physician, I had seen my share of suffering, but watching the patient decline was particularly harrowing. Their once hopeful demeanor faded, replaced by a weary acceptance of their fate. We transitioned to palliative care, aiming to provide comfort rather than cure. Pain management became a priority, alongside psychological support to help them cope with the emotional toll of their illness.

Throughout this ordeal, I often reflected on the nature of rare diseases like Caroli. The delayed diagnosis, the complex treatment strategies, and the inevitable complications highlighted the gaps in our medical knowledge and the limitations of our interventions. The patient's journey underscored the need for increased awareness and research into such conditions.

In the end, the patient's body could no longer endure the relentless assault of the disease and its complications. They passed away quietly, surrounded by family. Their struggle was over, but the memory of their courage and endurance remained with me. The lessons learned from their case informed my practice and deepened my understanding of the human aspect of medicine.

Caroli Disease had not been a familiar foe to me before, but it had left an indelible mark on my career and my perspective as a healer. The patient's story became a testament to the importance of vigilance, early diagnosis, and the compassionate care that every patient deserves, especially those battling rare and challenging conditions.

# CHAPTER NINE

## CHANARIN-DORFMAN SYNDROME

IT WAS an unremarkable Tuesday morning when I first encountered the patient who would forever alter my perspective on the intricate tapestry of human health. The early light filtered through the hospital blinds, casting long, slatted shadows across my desk. My morning rounds were typically predictable, a series of routine check-ups, follow-ups, and occasional emergency cases that broke the monotony. But this patient was different from the outset, their symptoms an enigmatic puzzle that would soon unravel into a diagnosis of Chanarin-Dorfman Syndrome, a rare and complex metabolic disorder.

The patient, a middle-aged individual of Mediterranean descent, had been referred to our department after presenting with a curious constellation of symptoms that had baffled their primary care physician. Upon their arrival, they exhibited signs of ichthyosis, a condition characterized by dry, scaly skin that glistened under the fluorescent lights of the examination room. There was something almost otherworldly about the way the scales caught the light, each flake a testament to the body's silent struggle against itself.

As I delved into their medical history, it became apparent that the patient had experienced a lifetime of seemingly unrelated health issues. There had been recurrent episodes of myopathy, muscle weakness that left them fatigued after even mild exertion. Liver function tests had consistently returned abnormal results, though previous investigations had failed to pinpoint a specific cause. The patient recounted episodes of unexplained abdominal pain and persistent diarrhea, symptoms that had been dismissed as irritable bowel syndrome for years. But it was the peculiar lipid droplets observed in a routine blood smear that had finally led to their referral to our clinic.

The initial physical examination was thorough. I noted the presence of hepatomegaly, the patient's liver palpable below the rib cage, firm and enlarged. This, coupled with the ichthyosis and muscle weakness, painted a picture that was both compelling and confounding. The next step was to order a battery of tests: liver function tests, creatine kinase levels, a complete blood count, and most crucially, a skin biopsy. The biopsy would confirm our suspicions by revealing lipid-laden vacuoles within the patient's cells, a hallmark of Chanarin-Dorfman Syndrome.

While waiting for the biopsy results, I pored over the existing literature on Chanarin-Dorfman Syndrome, a disorder so rare that it was often relegated to a footnote in medical textbooks. It was an autosomal recessive disorder, caused by mutations in the ABHD5 gene. This gene was responsible for encoding a protein essential for lipid metabolism. Without it, neutral lipids accumulated within various tissues, leading to the myriad symptoms the patient had endured.

The biopsy results confirmed our suspicions: lipid-laden vacuoles were present in the keratinocytes. The diagnosis was clear, but the path forward was anything but. Chanarin-Dorfman Syndrome was a chronic condition with no definitive cure, and treatment options were limited to managing symptoms and preventing complications.

We embarked on a comprehensive treatment plan, starting with dietary modifications to reduce lipid intake and alleviate the burden on the liver. A low-fat diet rich in medium-chain triglycerides was prescribed, designed to be more easily metabolized by the patient's compromised system. This dietary adjustment was not merely a suggestion but a cornerstone of their treatment, aimed at preventing further lipid accumulation.

In conjunction with dietary changes, we initiated a regimen of vitamin supplementation. Given the patient's ichthyosis, fat-soluble vitamins, particularly vitamin E, were administered to help mitigate the skin condition. Vitamin A was also prescribed cautiously, given its potential toxicity at high doses but essential role in maintaining skin health.

To address the myopathy, we introduced a physical therapy program tailored to the patient's needs. This program focused on strengthening the muscles without overexerting them, a delicate balance that required close monitoring and frequent adjustments. The physical therapist worked closely with the patient, guiding them through exercises that gradually increased in intensity as their strength improved.

The patient's liver function was closely monitored, and medications were prescribed to manage the associated symptoms. Ursodeoxycholic acid was introduced to help improve liver function and reduce the risk of cirrhosis. Regular blood tests were scheduled to track liver enzyme levels and adjust treatment as needed.

As weeks turned into months, the patient's condition began to stabilize. The dietary changes and vitamin supplementation had a noticeable impact on their skin, with the ichthyosis becoming less severe. The physical therapy program, while challenging, helped improve their muscle strength and endurance. The abdominal pain and diarrhea, though not completely resolved, became less frequent and severe.

However, the journey was far from linear. There were setbacks, moments when the patient's condition would deteriorate, and adjustments to the treatment plan were necessary. Infections became a frequent concern, as the patient's compromised immune system made them more susceptible. Each new infection was a reminder of the precarious balance we were striving to maintain.

Despite these challenges, the patient exhibited a remarkable tenacity. Their determination to adhere to the treatment plan, despite the numerous obstacles, was inspiring. They navigated each setback with a fortitude that spoke volumes about their character.

As the months progressed, the patient's quality of life improved incrementally. They reported increased energy levels, fewer episodes of abdominal pain, and a significant reduction in skin symptoms. These improvements, while modest, were victories in the context of a chronic, incurable condition.

Throughout this period, regular follow-ups became a

cornerstone of the treatment regimen. Each visit provided an opportunity to reassess the patient's condition, make necessary adjustments, and offer support and encouragement. The multidisciplinary team, including dietitians, physical therapists, and hepatologists, played a crucial role in managing the complex interplay of symptoms and treatments.

By the end of the first year, the patient's condition had reached a plateau. The symptoms were managed, if not entirely eliminated, and the patient's quality of life had improved significantly. The ichthyosis, once a glaring and painful symptom, had diminished to the point where it was manageable with routine skin care. Muscle strength had improved to the extent that the patient could engage in daily activities without debilitating fatigue. Liver function, while still abnormal, was stable, and the risk of complications had been reduced.

Despite these improvements, the reality of Chanarin-Dorfman Syndrome remained. It was a chronic condition, one that would require lifelong management and vigilance. The patient would need to adhere to their dietary restrictions, continue with physical therapy, and undergo regular monitoring to prevent and address complications promptly.

In the years that followed, the patient continued to manage their condition with the same unwavering determination. There were periods of stability punctuated by occasional setbacks, each navigated with the support of the medical team. The patient's journey with Chanarin-Dorfman Syndrome was a testament to the complex interplay between genetic destiny and the human spirit's indomitable strength.

# CHAPTER TEN

---

## DEXTROCARDIA WITH SITUS INVERSUS

WHEN I FIRST ENCOUNTERED THE patient, it was a typically busy Tuesday afternoon in the hospital. The air was thick with the scent of antiseptic, and the low hum of medical equipment filled the background as I went about my rounds. The patient was brought in by ambulance following a motor vehicle accident. They were a young adult, appearing in distress, with a myriad of cuts and bruises and a concerning level of chest pain. My initial assumption was that this pain was due to trauma from the collision, but the truth was far more intriguing and complex.

The paramedics had done a commendable job in stabilizing the patient and obtaining preliminary vitals. As I approached the stretcher, I noticed an unusual rhythm on the heart monitor—an electrical pattern that didn't quite fit the textbook examples of typical cardiac presentations. The patient's heart rate was elevated, but the peculiar placement of the leads seemed to indicate a deviation from the norm. I could not quite put my finger on it, but something seemed off.

With a calm yet urgent demeanor, I ordered a chest X-ray and an echocardiogram, suspecting internal injuries or a possible pneumothorax. The X-ray was the first to come back, and it left me momentarily perplexed. The heart shadow was on the right side of the thoracic cavity rather than the left. My initial thought was that the X-ray film might have been placed backward, a rare but not impossible clerical error. I requested a repeat of the X-ray to confirm my suspicions.

Meanwhile, I conducted a physical examination. The patient's breathing was labored, and their blood pressure was slightly elevated. I palpated the abdomen, checked for signs of internal bleeding, and listened to lung sounds. Every assessment indicated trauma, but the peculiarities of the heart placement could not be ignored. The second X-ray confirmed my initial observation—the heart was indeed situated on the right side of the chest cavity.

It was then that the echocardiogram results came in. The echocardiogram revealed that the patient had Dextrocardia with Situs Inversus, a rare congenital condition in which the heart is positioned on the right side of the body, and the organs in the abdomen and chest are mirrored from their normal positions. This diagnosis was unexpected, and it necessitated a swift adjustment in my approach to treatment. In a condition where every organ is a mirror image of the norm, surgical and diagnostic procedures must be recalibrated to avoid potentially catastrophic errors.

Dextrocardia with Situs Inversus is an uncommon congenital condition where the heart is a mirror image of its normal position, lying on the right side of the chest instead of the left. This condition is often accompanied by Situs Inversus, where the major visceral organs are reversed. The liver, typically on the right, is found on the left, the stomach on the right, and so forth. This condition can be part of a broader spectrum known as Kartagener's Syndrome, which also includes chronic sinusitis and bronchiectasis due to defective ciliary action in the respiratory tract.

The immediate concern was to manage the trauma resulting from the accident. The patient had sustained several rib fractures, and there was a minor hemothorax on the left side, which, under normal anatomical circumstances, would have been on the right. With the knowledge of the patient's Situs Inversus, the typical procedures were reversed. A chest tube was placed on the correct side to drain the accumulating blood and relieve pressure on the lungs.

Next, I ordered a full-body CT scan to assess any additional injuries and to get a comprehensive understanding of the internal layout. The CT scan further confirmed the mirrored anatomy—liver on the left, spleen on the right, and other organs similarly transposed. There were no signs of significant internal bleeding, which was a relief, but close monitoring was necessary due to the complex nature of the injuries and underlying condition.

Managing a patient with Dextrocardia with Situs Inversus presented a unique set of challenges. Routine procedures, such as placing central lines or performing emergency surgeries, required a mental re-mapping of the patient's anatomy. Medical staff had to be briefed and extra caution exercised to ensure that everyone was aware of the reversed organ positions. Despite the hectic environment, the team adapted quickly, demonstrating exceptional versatility and competence.

Throughout the patient's initial days in the Intensive Care Unit, I monitored their progress closely. Pain management was crucial, given the rib fractures and the chest tube placement. Analgesics were administered, and regular assessments ensured that the patient remained stable. There was a heightened risk of complications such as infection or pneumothorax recurrence, so vigilance was paramount.

As days turned into weeks, the patient began to show signs of improvement. The chest tube was eventually removed, and the fractures started to heal. Regular physiotherapy sessions were introduced to assist in regaining full respiratory function and mobility. The recovery process was slow but steady, each small milestone a testament to the patient's fortitude.

The patient's congenital condition necessitated a more thorough long-term management plan. Regular cardiac evaluations were scheduled to monitor heart health, as individuals with Dextrocardia are at a slightly higher risk of developing heart-related complications. Additionally, comprehensive documentation was created to inform any future medical professionals of the patient's unique anatomical layout, ensuring that any subsequent treatments would take this into account.

Dextrocardia with Situs Inversus can sometimes be accompanied by other congenital defects such as heart malformations. However, in this patient's case, the heart appeared structurally normal aside from its mirrored position. This was fortunate, as it meant there were no additional surgical interventions required beyond managing the trauma.

In the midst of these medical intricacies, I found

myself reflecting on the broader implications of this condition. Dextrocardia with Situs Inversus is a rare but not unheard-of anomaly, and it underscores the incredible diversity of human anatomy. Each patient presents a unique challenge, a puzzle to be solved with careful consideration and expertise. This case was a stark reminder of the importance of personalized medicine, where understanding the individual nuances of a patient's physiology can significantly impact the outcome of their treatment.

As the patient continued their recovery, their stamina was evident. They gradually transitioned from the ICU to a general ward, and then to outpatient care. Each step forward was a victory, a testament to their strength and the dedication of the medical team. Follow-up visits became less frequent as the patient regained their health and independence, though regular check-ups remained essential.

Throughout this journey, the patient's case became a point of discussion and learning within the hospital. It served as an educational experience for medical students and a reminder for seasoned professionals of the variability in human anatomy. The collaborative effort required to treat such a unique case fostered a deeper sense of camaraderie and professional respect among the staff.

In the end, the patient's recovery was a testament to modern medicine's capabilities and the human spirit's tenacity. While they would always carry the knowledge of their unique anatomy, it was ultimately just one part of their complex and multifaceted identity. Their experience highlighted the importance of adaptability, meticulous attention to detail, and the unwavering commitment to patient care that defines the medical profession.

---

# CHAPTER ELEVEN

THE PATIENT ARRIVED at my clinic on a foggy autumn morning, presenting with symptoms that had been troubling them for months. Their lips were tinged blue, a telltale sign of cyanosis, and they complained of persistent shortness of breath and fatigue. I noted their pale complexion and the clubbing of their fingers, signs that hinted at a chronic and severe underlying condition. As a cardiologist with years of experience, I had seen these symptoms before and knew they could signal a complex cardiovascular issue.

After a thorough examination, I ordered an echocardiogram, which revealed a heart defect. The patient had a ventricular septal defect (VSD) – a hole in the heart that allowed blood to flow between the left and right ventricles. This defect had gone undetected for years, leading to increased blood flow to the lungs and, ultimately, to pulmonary hypertension. Over time, the high pressure in the lungs had caused a reversal of the blood flow through the VSD, a phenomenon known as Eisenmenger syndrome. It was a grave diagnosis, and I felt a weight settle over me as I explained the condition to the patient.

Eisenmenger syndrome is a rare and severe complication of congenital heart disease, where long-standing pulmonary hypertension leads to the reversal of a left-to-right shunt to a right-to-left shunt. The prognosis varies, but without treatment, the condition is invariably progressive and often fatal. I explained that the primary goal of treatment would be to manage symptoms and prevent complications rather than cure the disease. Given the complexity of Eisenmenger syndrome, a multidisciplinary approach would be necessary.

The first step in managing the patient's condition was to stabilize their symptoms and improve their quality of life. I prescribed medications to reduce the pulmonary hypertension, including endothelin receptor antagonists and phosphodiesterase type 5 inhibitors. These drugs would help relax the blood vessels in the lungs, reducing the pressure and making it easier for the heart to pump blood. I also recommended supplemental oxygen therapy to alleviate the cyanosis and advised the patient to avoid strenuous activities that could exacerbate their symptoms.

Despite the medication, the patient's condition remained precarious. Eisenmenger syndrome is a delicate balancing act; too much exertion could lead to a sudden increase in pulmonary pressure, risking heart failure. Regular follow-ups were crucial to monitor their progress and adjust the treatment as necessary. Each visit, I assessed their oxygen levels, reviewed their symptoms, and performed additional echocardiograms to track any changes in their heart function.

Over the following months, the patient's symptoms stabilized somewhat, but they remained limited by their condition. Simple tasks like walking up a flight of stairs left them breathless and fatigued. The chronic hypoxia also took a toll on their overall health, leading to complications like secondary erythrocytosis – an increase in red blood cell production as the body tried to compensate for the low oxygen levels. This condition required periodic phlebotomies to reduce the risk of blood clots and strokes.

As time passed, the patient began to experience more frequent episodes of hemoptysis – coughing up blood, a sign of ruptured blood vessels in the lungs due to the high pressure. This development was alarming and necessitated more aggressive intervention. I consulted with a pulmonologist and a cardiothoracic surgeon to discuss potential treatment options. We considered the possibility of a heart-lung transplant, the only definitive cure for Eisenmenger syndrome, but the patient's overall health and the risks associated with such a complex surgery made them a less-than-ideal candidate.

Given the limited options, we focused on managing the hemoptysis and preventing further complications. The patient was admitted to the hospital multiple times for supportive care and blood transfusions when necessary. Each hospitalization was a stark reminder of the severity of their condition and the fragility of their health.

Throughout this period, the patient's spirit remained remarkable. They faced each setback with a determination that was both inspiring and heart-wrenching. Their family was a constant presence, providing support and encouragement during the darkest times. As a physician, witnessing the emotional toll on both the patient and their loved ones was one of the most challenging aspects of my job. It reinforced the importance of a holistic approach to care, addressing not only the physical but also the emotional and psychological needs of the patient.

The patient's condition continued to deteriorate

over the next few years. Despite our best efforts, the progression of Eisenmenger syndrome was relentless. They developed arrhythmias, irregular heartbeats that further complicated their treatment. We implanted a pacemaker to help regulate their heart rhythm, but it was only a temporary solution. The strain on their heart and lungs was becoming too great.

In the final stages of the disease, the patient's quality of life declined significantly. They became increasingly dependent on oxygen therapy and could no longer perform even the simplest tasks without assistance. The cyanosis deepened, and they experienced chronic fatigue and weakness. Palliative care became a primary focus, aiming to provide comfort and alleviate pain. We managed their symptoms with a combination of medications, including diuretics to reduce fluid buildup and opioids for pain relief.

Despite the inevitable outcome, the patient's strength of character never wavered. They expressed gratitude for the care they received and cherished the moments spent with their family. Their bravery in the face of such a devastating illness was a testament to the human spirit's capacity to endure.

In the end, the patient passed away peacefully, surrounded by their loved ones. It was a somber moment, but also a relief to know they were no longer suffering. As I reflected on their journey, I was reminded of the importance of compassion and empathy in medicine. Eisenmenger syndrome is a formidable adversary, but the patient's journey highlighted the resilience of the human spirit and the profound impact of supportive care.

Their story is one of courage and perseverance in the face of insurmountable odds. It serves as a reminder of the fragility of life and the importance of cherishing every moment. As a physician, it reinforced my commitment to providing compassionate care and the importance of a multidisciplinary approach in managing complex conditions like Eisenmenger syndrome. The patient's legacy lives on in the lessons learned and the lives touched by their remarkable journey.

# CHAPTER TWELVE

## DIAMOND-BLACKFAN ANEMIA

THE FIRST TIME I met the patient, it was a crisp morning in late autumn. The golden leaves swirled around the hospital entrance as I walked into the pediatric clinic. My schedule was packed that day, but one appointment stood out: a new case, a child presenting with fatigue and pallor. As a hematologist, I had seen my share of blood disorders, but nothing prepared me for what lay ahead with this patient.

Upon entering the examination room, I immediately noticed the patient's small stature and the waxy pallor that seemed to emanate from every pore. The parents, seated beside the examination table, wore expressions of deep concern. I began with a thorough history, noting that the patient had been unusually tired, struggled with physical activities, and often experienced shortness of breath. These symptoms had persisted despite a balanced diet and what seemed like adequate rest.

I proceeded with a physical examination, my hands gently probing for any tell-tale signs. The patient's skin felt cool and clammy, and I could palpate the liver edge easily, suggesting mild hepatomegaly. The spleen was also palpable, another red flag. Blood work was the next logical step, and I ordered a complete blood count (CBC) and a reticulocyte count, hoping these tests would shed some light on the underlying issue.

The results came back quickly. The CBC revealed a significantly low hemoglobin level, well below the normal range for a child of that age. The reticulocyte count was also low, indicating that the bone marrow was not producing enough new red blood cells. This combination pointed toward a form of anemia, but the exact type required further investigation. Given the severity of the findings, I decided to admit the patient for further testing and observation.

In the hospital, we conducted a bone marrow biopsy, which is the gold standard for diagnosing marrow-related disorders. The sample was sent to pathology, and while we waited for the results, I started the patient on a regimen of transfusions to stabilize the hemoglobin levels. Transfusions, while necessary, were only a temporary measure. We needed a definitive diagnosis to determine the best course of treatment.

The pathology report came back confirming my suspicions: the patient had Diamond-Blackfan Anemia (DBA), a rare congenital disorder characterized by the failure of the bone marrow to produce red blood cells. This diagnosis was both a relief and a new source of anxiety. Relief because we now knew what we were dealing with, and anxiety because DBA is a lifelong condition with no simple cure.

The treatment plan began with corticosteroids, the frontline therapy for DBA. Steroids can stimulate red blood cell production in some patients, providing a lifeline that reduces the need for frequent transfusions. The patient responded positively initially, with hemoglobin levels rising and physical symptoms abating. The improvement was heartening, but I remained cautious. Steroid therapy is a delicate balance; long-term use can lead to severe side effects, including growth suppression, osteoporosis, and increased susceptibility to infections.

As weeks turned into months, we monitored the patient's progress closely. Regular blood tests became a routine part of life, each one a moment of tense anticipation for the family. Despite the initial positive response, it soon became apparent that the patient was becoming steroid-dependent. The doses required to maintain normal hemoglobin levels were escalating, and the side effects began to manifest. The patient developed a round, puffy face characteristic of Cushing's syndrome, and there were early signs of growth retardation.

Given the diminishing returns of steroid therapy, we explored other options. Hematopoietic stem cell transplantation (HSCT) was the next consideration. HSCT is the only potential cure for DBA, involving the transplantation of healthy stem cells to replace the defective marrow. However, this procedure carries significant risks, including graft-versus-host disease (GVHD) and other complications associated with high-dose chemotherapy used to prepare the body for the new stem cells.

Finding a suitable donor proved challenging. Siblings are often the best match, but the patient was an only child. We turned to the national bone marrow registry, casting a wide net in the hope of finding a compatible donor. Meanwhile, we also started the patient on an iron chelation therapy to counteract the iron overload from frequent blood transfusions. Iron overload can damage vital organs, particularly the heart and liver, so managing it was critical.

The search for a donor dragged on for months, during which time the patient's condition remained stable but precarious. Eventually, a partial match was found, and after extensive deliberation with the family, we proceeded with the transplant. The preparation phase was grueling. High-dose chemotherapy ravaged the patient's body, leading to hair loss, severe nausea, and a compromised immune system. The actual transplant, a simple transfusion of stem cells, was anticlimactic compared to the buildup.

Post-transplant, the patient was placed in isolation to protect against infections while the new marrow took hold. This period was fraught with tension. Every fever spike, every cough, was scrutinized and treated aggressively. The patient's resilience during this phase was remarkable. Despite the discomfort and the sterile isolation, there was a quiet determination that shone through the fatigue.

Weeks turned into months, and slowly, the new stem cells began to produce healthy red blood cells. The first signs of engraftment were met with cautious optimism. As the patient's counts stabilized, we began the gradual process of tapering off the immunosuppressive drugs that had been protecting the new marrow from being rejected. Each clinic visit revealed incremental improvements – a slightly higher hemoglobin here, a stable white cell count there. It was progress, albeit slow and fraught with setbacks.

Complications were inevitable. The patient developed mild GVHD, manifesting as a skin rash and gastrointestinal symptoms. We managed these with a careful balance of medications, constantly adjusting to keep the symptoms under control without compromising the new marrow. The months following the transplant were a delicate dance of monitoring, adjusting, and hoping.

As the first year post-transplant drew to a close, the patient showed remarkable improvement. The need for transfusions had ceased, and the hemoglobin levels remained within normal limits. The corticosteroid-induced side effects began to reverse, with the patient's face returning to a more normal contour and signs of growth resuming, albeit slowly. There were still challenges ahead – regular follow-ups, potential long-term effects of the treatment, and the psychological impact of such an intense medical journey.

The journey was long and arduous, marked by highs and lows, victories and setbacks. The patient, through every stage, demonstrated a quiet strength and tenacity that was deeply moving. For a child to endure such a relentless assault on their body and spirit and come out the other side with a smile was nothing short of inspirational. The family's unwavering support and faith played a crucial role, providing a bedrock of love and stability amidst the chaos of treatment.

In the end, the transplant was deemed a success.

The patient's marrow continued to produce healthy blood cells, and the episodes of GVHD became less frequent and severe. The patient's life, while not without its medical complexities, began to assume a semblance of normalcy. Regular school attendance, play-dates, and the simple joys of childhood that had been overshadowed by illness slowly returned.

Throughout this journey, I learned as much from the patient as I hope they did from my care. The intricate dance of medical science and human spirit was on full display, reminding me of the profound impact of compassion, perseverance, and hope. Every time I saw the patient's name on my clinic list, it was a reminder of the resilience of the human body and spirit, and the incredible power of hope in the face of daunting odds.

My role as a doctor in this journey was part healer, part guide, and part witness to an incredible story of survival and determination. The patient's story will stay with me always, a testament to the indomitable will to live and the miracles of modern medicine.

# CHAPTER THIRTEEN

## CASTLEMAN DISEASE

AS A PHYSICIAN, I've encountered myriad illnesses, but few cases left as indelible a mark on my memory as that of the patient with Castleman disease. The patient first came to my attention during a routine physical examination, a picture of subtle malaise that belied the storm brewing within.

It started with the patient reporting generalized weakness and fatigue, symptoms that were deceptively mundane and easily attributed to the stresses of daily life. Yet, there was something in the patient's eyes—a weary resignation that spoke of a deeper, unspoken torment. A detailed history and physical examination were warranted. I noted the patient's weight loss, a significant 10% decrease over three months, and mild splenomegaly upon abdominal palpation. The lymph nodes were barely palpable, yet firm, and slightly tender in the cervical and axillary regions.

Routine blood tests initially suggested an inflammatory process: elevated erythrocyte sedimentation rate (ESR) and C-reactive protein (CRP). However, these markers alone were nonspecific and required further exploration. The differential diagnosis ranged from infectious causes to autoimmune disorders. As the symptoms persisted, I ordered a comprehensive workup, including imaging studies.

A contrast-enhanced CT scan of the chest, abdomen, and pelvis revealed multiple enlarged lymph nodes, particularly in the mediastinum and retroperitoneum. The patient's liver and spleen were also slightly enlarged, raising concerns about a possible underlying hematologic malignancy. I recommended an excisional biopsy of one of the more accessible lymph nodes to get a clearer picture.

The pathology report confirmed Castleman disease, specifically the multicentric variant. This was a rare and complex lymphoproliferative disorder characterized by systemic inflammation and multiple organ involvement. I explained the diagnosis to the patient, focusing on the nature of the disease, its potential complications, and the treatment options available.

The patient's treatment plan required a multidisciplinary approach, involving oncologists, hematologists, and infectious disease specialists. We initiated therapy with corticosteroids to reduce the inflammation and control symptoms. However, the patient's condition did not improve significantly, necessitating the addition of more aggressive therapies.

The next line of treatment was rituximab, a monoclonal antibody targeting the CD20 protein on B cells. This approach was chosen due to its efficacy in other lymphoproliferative disorders and its ability to deplete the aberrant B cell population driving the disease. The patient tolerated the infusions well initially, but soon developed infusion-related reactions, including fever, chills, and hypotension. These side effects were managed with premedication and supportive care, allowing the patient to complete the course of therapy.

Despite these interventions, the patient's disease showed only partial response. We proceeded to administer siltuximab, another monoclonal antibody, but one that specifically targets interleukin-6 (IL-6), a cytokine implicated in the pathogenesis of Castleman disease. Siltuximab was given every three weeks, and this time, we observed a more pronounced reduction in lymph node size and improvement in systemic symptoms.

Throughout the treatment, the patient displayed remarkable fortitude. The fatigue that once plagued the patient began to diminish, and weight stabilized. Regular follow-ups showed a gradual normalization of inflammatory markers and improvement in organ function. Yet, the road to remission was not without its hurdles. The patient's immunosuppressed state led to several opportunistic infections, including a severe bout of pneumocystis pneumonia that required hospitalization and intravenous antibiotics.

The infectious disease team worked diligently to manage these complications, providing prophylactic antibiotics and antifungals to prevent further episodes. Additionally, the patient's nutritional status needed constant monitoring, as the disease and its treatment took a toll on their appetite and gastrointestinal function. We employed a comprehensive nutrition plan, including supplements and parenteral nutrition when necessary, to maintain the patient's strength and support recovery.

As months turned into a year, the patient remained under close surveillance. Imaging studies continued to show stable disease, with no new lymphadenopathy or organomegaly. The patient gradually returned to a semblance of normalcy, resuming activities that had been forsaken due to illness.

However, Castleman disease is known for its potential to relapse, and so we maintained a cautious optimism. The patient was transitioned to maintenance therapy with low-dose corticosteroids and regular follow-ups to monitor for any signs of recurrence. The specter of relapse loomed, but for the time being, the patient was in remission.

In the following years, the patient continued to navigate life with the ever-present awareness of their condition. Routine check-ups became a part of their new normal, each one a small victory in the ongoing battle against Castleman disease. The patient adhered to the maintenance therapy regimen with diligence, knowing that vigilance was their strongest ally.

Unfortunately, the precarious balance was disrupted two years after the initial remission. During a routine visit, the patient reported feeling increasingly fatigued and experiencing night sweats. Blood tests revealed elevated inflammatory markers, and a subsequent CT scan confirmed our fears: there was new lymphadenopathy in the mediastinum and abdomen, alongside splenomegaly.

We resumed more intensive treatment, this time combining rituximab with chemotherapy. The patient's resilience was tested anew as they endured the side effects of the treatment: nausea, hair loss, and profound fatigue. Despite these challenges, the patient faced each day with quiet determination.

The chemotherapy regimen led to a partial response,

reducing the size of the lymph nodes but not achieving complete remission. It was clear that Castleman disease was proving to be refractory. At this juncture, we decided to enroll the patient in a clinical trial for a new targeted therapy aimed at disrupting the specific pathways involved in Castleman disease.

The patient received the investigational drug as part of the trial protocol, monitored closely for both efficacy and adverse effects. Initial results were promising: the lymph nodes shrank, and the patient experienced a marked improvement in symptoms. However, this period of improvement was transient. Six months into the trial, the patient developed severe cytopenias, a side effect of the new drug, which necessitated discontinuation of the treatment.

With options dwindling, we turned to supportive care and symptom management, focusing on maintaining the patient's quality of life. The interdisciplinary team included palliative care specialists who provided pain management, psychological support, and advanced care planning.

As the disease progressed, the patient became more reliant on caregivers. They faced each day with unwavering courage, finding solace in small pleasures and the company of loved ones. Their strength in the face of such an overwhelming illness was nothing short of inspiring.

Ultimately, Castleman disease claimed the patient's life. The final stages were marked by organ failure, a consequence of the relentless systemic inflammation and multiorgan involvement characteristic of the disease. The patient passed away surrounded by family, their battle with Castleman disease leaving a lasting impact on all who witnessed it.

Reflecting on the patient's journey, I am reminded of the complexity and unpredictability of Castleman disease. The initial diagnosis, the series of treatments, and the eventual outcome underscore the challenges in managing this rare condition. Each step of the way, the patient's indomitable spirit shone through, a testament to human strength in the face of adversity.

The patient's case remains a poignant example of the need for continued research and advancements in the treatment of rare diseases. While we were able to extend life and improve the quality of life for a period, the ultimate goal remains a cure. Until that day comes, we as physicians must continue to strive for the best possible outcomes for our patients, offering them hope and support through every stage of their journey.

# CHAPTER FOURTEEN

## REDWATER FEVER

IT WAS the hottest summer I could remember, and the relentless sun bore down on our small clinic in the heart of the delta. The air was thick with humidity, and the scent of magnolia blossoms mixed with the brackish aroma of the nearby river. It was a time when the seasons seemed to blur into one another, marked only by the cyclical rhythm of life and death in our isolated community.

On one particularly stifling afternoon, the patient arrived, carried in by a worried family member. They had traveled far, through sweltering heat and dense thickets, to reach our modest facility. The patient's condition was dire; the skin was flushed, and beads of sweat dotted their forehead. As I laid eyes on them, I knew immediately that this was no ordinary case. The telltale signs were all too familiar to me: a deep crimson hue to the skin, eyes that seemed to burn with fever, and a palpable sense of distress.

My mind raced through the possibilities, but one diagnosis stood out among the rest – Redwater Fever. This insidious disease, transmitted by the bite of the Anopheles mosquito, had a reputation for ravaging the body with an unyielding grip. Its onset was sudden, and its effects could be devastating. As a physician in this remote region, I had encountered it before, but each case was unique, each patient's struggle a testament to the human spirit's capacity for endurance.

The first step was to confirm the diagnosis. I ordered a blood test, knowing that the presence of the Plasmodium parasite would reveal the truth. The results came back swiftly, and my suspicions were confirmed. The patient was indeed suffering from Redwater Fever. The parasite had invaded their red blood cells, causing them to rupture and releasing toxins into their bloodstream. This explained the deep red hue of their skin – a macabre signature of the disease.

Treatment had to be immediate and aggressive. Redwater Fever was not something that could be managed with half measures. I began with a high dose of quinine, the most effective antimalarial we had at our disposal. The bitter liquid was administered through an intravenous drip, its potent properties coursing through the patient's veins. Quinine, though effective, came with its own set of challenges. Its side effects could be harsh – ringing in the ears, nausea, and even vision disturbances – but it was our best hope.

I monitored the patient's vital signs closely, noting every fluctuation in temperature, heart rate, and blood pressure. The fever raged on, relentless in its assault. Each spike in temperature was a battle, and I fought back with cold compresses and antipyretics. The patient shivered uncontrollably despite the oppressive heat, their body wracked with chills. It was a cruel paradox – burning with fever yet trembling with cold.

Days turned into nights, and I seldom left the patient's side. Sleep was a luxury I could not afford; my duty was to this individual who lay before me, fighting for their life. The clinic, usually a place of quiet routine, had become a battlefield. The buzzing of mosquitoes outside served as a constant reminder of the unseen enemy we were up against.

As the treatment progressed, I noticed a slight improvement. The fever, once a raging inferno, began to subside. The patient's skin, though still unnaturally red, had lost some of its alarming intensity. The quinine was working, attacking the parasite within the blood cells, but the battle was far from over. The patient's body had been weakened, their immune system compromised by the relentless onslaught.

Hydration was critical. The toxins released by the ruptured blood cells needed to be flushed out, and so I administered intravenous fluids to prevent dehydration. The patient, too weak to consume much orally, accepted the drip with a weary nod. Electrolyte imbalances had to be corrected, and I carefully monitored their levels, adjusting the fluids as necessary.

Nutrition posed another challenge. The patient's appetite was nonexistent, their body rejecting even the simplest of foods. I resorted to nutrient-rich broths and, when necessary, supplemental feeding through a nasogastric tube. The patient's weight had dropped alarmingly, their once robust frame now gaunt and frail. Each day was a struggle to maintain their strength, to provide the body with the energy it needed to fight the parasite and begin the slow process of healing.

Complications were inevitable. The prolonged fever had taken its toll on the patient's liver and kidneys, organs already stressed by the parasitic infection. Jaundice set in, the whites of their eyes turning a sickly yellow. I adjusted the treatment regimen, adding medications to support liver function and increase urine output. It was a delicate balance – too much intervention, and the body could be overwhelmed; too little, and the organs could fail.

Despite the mounting challenges, there were moments of hope. The patient's breathing, once labored and shallow, began to steady. The heart, though still working hard, showed signs of stabilizing. I clung to these small victories, using them as fuel to press on. The patient's will to live was evident, even in their weakened state. It was a silent determination, a resolve that mirrored my own.

As the days passed, the patient entered a critical phase. The fever had broken, but the road to recovery was fraught with obstacles. The damage done by the parasite was extensive, and the body needed time to repair itself. The patient's strength returned slowly, each day bringing a slight improvement. Their skin, once an angry red, began to regain a more natural hue, though the underlying weakness remained.

Physical therapy became an integral part of the recovery process. Muscles that had atrophied from prolonged bed rest needed to be strengthened. Simple exercises, once taken for granted, became milestones – the ability to sit up unaided, to stand, to take a few tentative steps. It was a slow and arduous journey, but each small triumph was a step toward a semblance of normalcy.

Emotionally, the toll of the illness was profound. The patient had been to the brink of death and back, and the psychological scars were deep. Nightmares plagued their sleep, memories of fevered hallucinations mingling with reality. I offered what comfort I could, a steady presence in a world that had been turned upside down. The support of the patient's family was invaluable, their unwavering faith and love providing a foundation upon which to rebuild.

Weeks turned into months, and the patient continued to improve. The once gaunt frame began to fill out, strength returning to limbs that had been frail and weak. The jaundice faded, the liver and kidneys slowly regaining their function. Blood tests showed a decreasing presence of the parasite, a sign that the treatment had been successful.

Despite the progress, the patient would never be the same. Redwater Fever had left its mark, a reminder of the fragility of life in this unforgiving land. The body had been scarred, the organs taxed beyond their limits, but the patient had survived. It was a testament to the human spirit's tenacity, the will to fight even in the face of overwhelming odds.

The journey had been long and arduous, a battle fought on multiple fronts. As a physician, I had been both a guide and a witness to this struggle. The experience had deepened my understanding of the delicate balance between life and death, the thin line that separates survival from defeat.

In the end, it was not just the medicine that had made the difference, but the patient's own unyielding spirit, their ability to endure, to fight, to survive. The clinic, once a place of quiet routine, had become a battlefield where life triumphed over the shadow of death. And as the patient took their first steps out of the clinic, supported by their loved ones, I felt a deep sense of gratitude. It was a reminder of why I had chosen this path, of the profound impact that one life can have, and the enduring strength of the human spirit.

# CHAPTER FIFTEEN

## WALDENSTRÖM MACROGLOBULINEMIA

THE PATIENT ARRIVED at my clinic with a persistent fatigue that had gradually worsened over the past several months. This wasn't uncommon; many of my patients came to me with vague symptoms like tiredness, which could be attributed to countless benign causes. However, I sensed something more sinister lurking beneath the surface as I examined the patient.

The physical examination was unremarkable at first, with no immediate signs of illness. Yet, the patient's pallor and slight weight loss hinted at an underlying issue. I ordered a battery of tests, including a complete blood count and a comprehensive metabolic panel. When the results returned, they revealed an elevated erythrocyte sedimentation rate and a high level of serum protein. These findings, though nonspecific, suggested an inflammatory or neoplastic process. Further investigation was warranted.

I proceeded with serum protein electrophoresis, a test used to detect abnormal proteins in the blood. The results showed a monoclonal protein spike, indicating the presence of a monoclonal gammopathy. The patient was then subjected to a bone marrow biopsy, a more invasive procedure but crucial for a definitive diagnosis. The biopsy revealed an infiltration of lymphoplasmacytic cells, confirming my suspicion of Waldenström Macroglobulinemia, a rare type of non-Hodgkin lymphoma.

The diagnosis of Waldenström Macroglobulinemia often comes as a shock, both to the patient and to their family. It is a chronic, indolent disease characterized by the production of abnormal monoclonal immunoglobulin M (IgM) protein. This protein thickens the blood, leading to a range of symptoms, including fatigue, neuropathy, and hyperviscosity syndrome. Understanding the disease's nature and potential progression is vital for planning the patient's treatment.

The initial step in managing Waldenström Macroglobulinemia involves addressing the hyperviscosity. Plasmapheresis was the immediate intervention, a process that filters the blood to reduce the level of IgM. The patient tolerated this procedure well, experiencing immediate relief from some of the more debilitating symptoms, such as headaches and dizziness.

Following plasmapheresis, the next phase of treatment aimed at targeting the underlying malignancy. Given the patient's overall good health and absence of significant comorbidities, I recommended a combination therapy of rituximab and bendamustine. Rituximab, a monoclonal antibody, targets the CD20 antigen on the surface of B-cells, while bendamustine, a chemotherapeutic agent, disrupts the DNA in cancer cells, leading to their death.

Chemotherapy is a double-edged sword, often causing as much harm as good. The patient endured the common side effects of nausea, fatigue, and hair loss with a remarkable fortitude. Despite these challenges, regular follow-ups and blood tests showed a gradual decline in the IgM levels, indicating that the treatment was effective.

Throughout this journey, managing the complications of both the disease and its treatment was crucial. The patient developed peripheral neuropathy, a common side effect of rituximab, resulting in numbness and tingling in the extremities. Gabapentin was prescribed to alleviate these symptoms. Additionally, the patient experienced bouts of anemia and required periodic blood transfusions to maintain adequate hemoglobin levels.

One of the most challenging aspects of treating Waldenström Macroglobulinemia is the disease's unpredictable course. While some patients achieve long-term remission, others may experience a relapse. Regular monitoring through blood tests and imaging studies is essential to detect any signs of disease progression early.

Months passed, and the patient responded well to the initial therapy. The IgM levels stabilized, and the symptoms were under control. However, this period of stability was marred by an unexpected development. During a routine follow-up, the patient reported new symptoms of abdominal discomfort and early satiety. An ultrasound revealed splenomegaly, an enlargement of the spleen, a complication that can arise due to the infiltration of malignant cells.

Given this new complication, I decided to initiate a second line of treatment. Ibrutinib, a Bruton's tyrosine kinase (BTK) inhibitor, was introduced. Ibrutinib works by blocking the signals that promote the survival and proliferation of B-cells. This targeted therapy offered hope, as it had shown promise in patients with relapsed or refractory Waldenström Macroglobulinemia.

The patient began the new treatment regimen, and within weeks, there was a noticeable improvement in the symptoms. The spleen size reduced, and the abdominal discomfort subsided. However, the therapy was not without its side effects. The patient experienced episodes of diarrhea and mild bleeding, complications that were managed with supportive care and dose adjustments.

Throughout this arduous journey, the patient exhibited a remarkable fortitude. The battle against Waldenström Macroglobulinemia is often long and fraught with challenges. The support from family and a dedicated healthcare team played a pivotal role in navigating this complex landscape.

As months turned into years, the patient continued to show a favorable response to the treatment. Regular monitoring remained essential, with periodic blood tests and imaging studies to track the disease's status. The patient's life, though altered by the diagnosis, regained a semblance of normalcy. Engaging in daily activities, spending time with loved ones, and finding joy in small moments became possible again.

Despite the progress, the specter of relapse loomed large. Waldenström Macroglobulinemia is a chronic condition, and the potential for disease recurrence is a reality that patients and their doctors must face. The goal is to achieve the longest possible remission, with a focus on maintaining quality of life.

The patient experienced several more years of stability, a testament to the advancements in targeted therapies and the power of early intervention. However, in the seventh year following the initial diagnosis, signs of relapse emerged. The IgM levels began to rise, and the patient experienced fatigue and neuropathy once again.

At this juncture, a new treatment strategy was required. Zanubrutinib, another BTK inhibitor, was introduced. This newer generation of targeted therapy offered hope for prolonged remission. The patient started on this treatment with cautious optimism, aware of the journey's unpredictable nature.

The introduction of zanubrutinib brought renewed hope. The patient's symptoms gradually improved, and the IgM levels stabilized once more. Regular follow-ups and supportive care continued to be essential components of the treatment plan.

Over the next several years, the patient's condition remained stable. The advancements in medical research and the availability of newer therapies played a crucial role in managing the disease effectively. The patient's life, though shadowed by the constant presence of Waldenström Macroglobulinemia, was marked by moments of joy and fulfillment.

As a physician, witnessing the patient's journey through the highs and lows of this chronic illness was a profound experience. The determination and strength exhibited by the patient were a testament to the human spirit's capacity to endure and thrive despite adversity.

Waldenström Macroglobulinemia, with its chronic nature and potential for relapse, demands a vigilant and adaptive approach to treatment. The patient's story exemplifies the importance of early diagnosis, effective management, and the continuous pursuit of advancements in medical research to improve outcomes for those affected by this rare disease.

# CHAPTER SIXTEEN

## UPPER TRACT UROTHELIAL CARCINOMA

UPPER TRACT UROTHELIAL CARCINOMA, a rare and aggressive form of cancer, often presents a daunting challenge for both the patient and the medical team. I had encountered it numerous times throughout my career, yet each case retained its unique imprint on my memory. The patient arrived at my clinic with vague symptoms, typical of this elusive disease. It began, as it often does, with hematuria—blood in the urine—a symptom that is often ignored or misattributed until it becomes too persistent to overlook.

The patient's initial consultation was routine, marked by a nonchalant attitude common among those unaware of the storm brewing within them. A urine test confirmed the presence of microscopic hematuria, a sign I knew could not be dismissed. Given the patient's history and risk factors—age, smoking, and previous occupational exposure to certain chemicals—I recommended further investigation. The initial ultrasound scan revealed a mass in the renal pelvis, a discovery that necessitated a more detailed examination.

A CT urogram was performed, providing a clearer image of the mass. It was irregular, enhancing with contrast, suggestive of malignancy. The patient remained stoic as I explained the need for a ureteroscopy and biopsy, procedures essential for obtaining a definitive diagnosis. These tests would determine the nature of the growth and guide our next steps.

During the ureteroscopy, a flexible scope was inserted through the urethra, bladder, and up into the ureter. The mass was visible, its irregular surface ominously hinting at its malignant nature. Biopsy samples were taken, and a few days later, the pathology report confirmed our fears: high-grade upper tract urothelial carcinoma. The cancer cells were aggressive, prone to rapid growth and spread.

With the diagnosis in hand, we discussed the treatment options. Radical nephroureterectomy, the surgical removal of the kidney, ureter, and a cuff of the bladder, was the recommended approach for such an aggressive tumor. The patient listened quietly, absorbing the gravity of the situation. The decision to proceed with surgery was made, driven by the understanding that this offered the best chance for survival.

The surgery was scheduled promptly. It was a complex procedure, involving meticulous dissection to ensure clear margins and minimize the risk of recurrence. The patient's recovery was closely monitored, each day a testament to the human body's capacity to heal. Pain management, prevention of infections, and gradual reintroduction of physical activity were carefully balanced.

Post-operative scans and regular cystoscopies became routine, vigilance a necessary ally in the fight against cancer. The patient underwent adjuvant chemotherapy to address any microscopic residual disease. The side effects were severe: nausea, fatigue, and a profound sense of malaise. Yet, through it all, the patient's demeanor remained steadfast, a quiet determination evident in their eyes.

Months turned into years, each follow-up appointment a small victory. The scans remained clear, and no evidence of disease recurrence was detected. The patient resumed a semblance of normalcy, returning to work and engaging in activities once taken for granted. The shadow of cancer lingered, but it no longer dominated their existence.

Yet, the story did not end there. Three years post-surgery, a routine scan revealed an anomaly. A small, enhancing lesion in the bladder, suspicious for recurrence. A biopsy confirmed it: urothelial carcinoma had returned, this time in the bladder. The recurrence was a cruel reminder of the insidious nature of cancer, its ability to lurk undetected, waiting for the opportune moment to strike again.

Intravesical BCG therapy was initiated, a treatment involving the instillation of a live but weakened bacterium directly into the bladder. The aim was to provoke a local immune response against the cancer cells. The therapy was grueling, each session a test of endurance. Side effects included a burning sensation during urination, frequent urges to urinate, and flu-like symptoms.

Despite these challenges, the patient endured, buoyed by the hope that this treatment would eradicate the cancer. Follow-up cystoscopies showed initial success, the lesion shrinking in size. However, the battle was far from over. Multiple cycles of BCG were required, each one a reminder of the precarious balance between health and disease.

The years that followed were marked by a cautious optimism. The patient remained under close surveillance, regular scans and cystoscopies a part of their new normal. The psychological toll of living under the constant threat of recurrence was immense. Anxiety before each follow-up, the dread of hearing the words "It's back," weighed heavily on both of us.

Despite the frequent medical interventions and the psychological burden, the patient's spirit never wavered. They continued to live their life with a sense of purpose, finding solace in small joys and the support of loved ones. The periodic clean scans were celebrated quietly, each one a testament to their tenacity and the effectiveness of the treatment regimen.

As the years passed, the intervals between follow-ups increased, a sign of growing confidence in the patient's long-term prognosis. The threat of recurrence never completely dissipated, but it became a background hum rather than a deafening roar. The patient had learned to coexist with the uncertainty, a skill that few master but many must endure.

Eventually, a decade passed since the initial diagnosis. The patient remained cancer-free, a milestone that marked a significant achievement in their journey. The medical community often measures success in five-year survival rates, but in cases like these, every year, every clean scan, is a triumph.

The story of the patient is one of countless tales in the annals of oncology. Each journey through cancer is unique, shaped by individual responses to treatment, personal resilience, and the unpredictable nature of the disease. As a physician, bearing witness to such journeys is both a privilege and a profound responsibility. The patient's courage and tenacity were a reminder of the indomitable will to live, an inspiration that transcended the clinical setting.

While the battle against upper tract urothelial carcinoma was fraught with challenges, the patient's story serves as a beacon of hope. It underscores the importance of early detection, the efficacy of combined treatment modalities, and the critical role of ongoing surveillance in managing this aggressive cancer. Their journey, marked by determination and endurance, continues to inspire those who face similar battles, a testament to the resilience of the human spirit.

# CHAPTER SEVENTEEN

## SAETHRE CHOTZEN SYNDROME

SAETHRE-CHOTZEN SYNDROME, a rare craniosynostosis syndrome, entered my professional life through a case that would forever shape my understanding of courage and vulnerability. I remember the day the patient was admitted as if it were yesterday. They were a young child, barely past their fifth birthday, brought in by worried parents who had noticed some irregularities in their child's skull shape and development. The patient's forehead appeared unusually prominent, and their eyes were set wider apart than normal. There was also a noticeable asymmetry to the face, and their fingers seemed shorter, almost fused.

The initial visit was fraught with anxiety. The parents had consulted their pediatrician, who had referred them to us after noting the irregularities. My role as a nurse was to assist in the diagnostic process and provide comfort and information to the family. I knew this would be a complex journey, both medically and emotionally.

The first step was a thorough physical examination. The pediatrician and craniofacial specialist noted the characteristic features of Saethre-Chotzen Syndrome, a condition caused by mutations in the TWIST1 gene. To confirm the diagnosis, genetic testing was necessary. I remember holding the patient's hand as a small blood sample was taken, their tiny fingers gripping mine tightly. The genetic test confirmed our suspicions. The mutation in the TWIST1 gene was present, and the diagnosis was clear.

Explaining the condition to the parents was a delicate task. They were overwhelmed, bombarded with a flood of medical terminology and possible outcomes. I spent a significant amount of time with them, breaking down the information into manageable parts, providing pamphlets and diagrams, and answering their myriad questions. I could see the fear in their eyes, the uncertainty of what the future held for their child.

The next phase involved planning the course of treatment. Saethre-Chotzen Syndrome often requires surgical intervention to correct the craniosynostosis and prevent further complications. The craniofacial team, including surgeons, anesthetists, and pediatricians, convened to discuss the patient's case. It was decided that cranial vault remodeling surgery would be necessary. This surgery would correct the premature fusion of the cranial sutures, allowing the brain to grow and develop properly, and address the cosmetic concerns that could impact the patient's quality of life.

The day of the surgery was filled with a tense anticipation. As a nurse, I was part of the pre-operative team, preparing the patient and providing reassurance to the parents. The patient was remarkably calm, displaying a sense of quiet strength that belied their age. I carefully explained the procedures we were performing, from the insertion of the intravenous line to the application of monitoring devices, making sure the patient felt safe and informed.

The surgery itself was a lengthy and complex procedure. I remained in the operating room, assisting where needed and monitoring the patient's vitals. The craniofacial surgeon meticulously worked to reshape the patient's skull, carefully separating the fused sutures and repositioning the bones. It was a delicate balance of skill and precision, every movement calculated and deliberate. The hours ticked by slowly, each one bringing us closer to the hopeful conclusion that the patient would emerge from this ordeal with a brighter future.

Post-operatively, the patient was transferred to the pediatric intensive care unit for close monitoring. The first 24 hours were critical, with the risk of swelling and complications looming large. I stayed by the patient's bedside, monitoring vital signs, administering medications, and providing comfort. The patient's face was swollen, bandages wrapping their head, but there was a sense of peace in their slumber. The parents, though anxious, were reassured by the constant care and updates provided by our team.

Recovery was a gradual process. The swelling subsided over the next few days, and the patient began to wake, disoriented but otherwise stable. Pain management was a priority, and we employed a combination of medications to keep the patient comfortable. The first time the patient opened their eyes and recognized their parents, there was an overwhelming sense of relief. Their parents held their child's hands, tears streaming down their faces, and I felt a deep sense of privilege to witness this moment.

The patient's stay in the hospital extended over several weeks. During this time, we focused not only on physical recovery but also on the psychological and developmental aspects. Physical therapy was introduced to help with any motor skills impacted by the surgery, and occupational therapy sessions began to address any challenges in fine motor skills and daily activities. I worked closely with the therapists, ensuring the patient's progress was meticulously tracked and any concerns were promptly addressed.

As the days turned into weeks, the patient's strength grew. There were moments of frustration and pain, but also moments of triumph and joy. The first time the patient smiled after the surgery was a milestone. That simple act signaled not just physical healing but a return to the joyful spirit that had been momentarily dimmed by the medical ordeal.

Regular follow-up appointments became a routine part of the patient's life. These visits allowed us to monitor their progress and address any emerging concerns. The craniofacial team was dedicated to ensuring the best possible outcomes, and this included considering further surgeries as the patient grew. Adjustments and refinements were sometimes necessary to accommodate the natural growth and changes that occur during childhood.

One of the significant challenges was addressing the psychological impact of having a rare genetic condition. The patient's parents were diligent in seeking support, enrolling their child in a support group for families dealing with craniofacial anomalies. This provided a sense of community and understanding, a space where the patient could interact with others who shared similar experiences. I encouraged this involvement, knowing the value of social and emotional support in the healing process.

School posed its own set of challenges. The patient faced curiosity and, at times, unkindness from peers who didn't understand their condition. The school staff was supportive, implementing educational programs to foster understanding and acceptance among the students. I worked with the family to develop strategies to navigate these social dynamics, emphasizing the importance of confidence and self-acceptance.

As years passed, the patient grew into a resilient and self-assured individual. They faced additional surgeries and medical interventions with a bravery that was nothing short of remarkable. Each procedure brought its own set of challenges, but also progress and improvement. The patient's craniofacial structure became more symmetrical, and the associated complications of the syndrome were managed effectively through ongoing medical care.

Throughout this journey, I remained involved, a constant presence in the patient's medical team. Watching the patient transition from a vulnerable child to a strong and confident young individual was one of the most rewarding experiences of my career. The bond formed with the patient and their family was profound, built on trust, empathy, and mutual respect.

In the end, the patient emerged not just as a survivor of Saethre-Chotzen Syndrome but as an individual who faced immense challenges with a steadfast spirit. Their journey continues, with regular medical check-ups and the occasional surgical intervention, but their story is one of courage and perseverance. As a nurse, I am honored to have been part of this journey, to have witnessed the patient's transformation and to have contributed to their care.

# CHAPTER EIGHTEEN

## COXIELLOSIS

THE PATIENT WAS a middle-aged man who had been living on a small farm on the outskirts of town. His initial symptoms were subtle—mild fever, headaches, and muscle aches—that could easily be mistaken for a common viral infection. When he first came to my clinic, I thought little of it. It was late summer, and such symptoms were common among farmers who spent long hours working in the heat. I advised rest, hydration, and a follow-up if the symptoms persisted. Little did I know that this was just the beginning of a much more serious condition.

A week later, the patient returned, looking worse than before. His fever had intensified, and he now complained of severe headaches and a dry cough. He mentioned that his muscle aches had turned into sharp pains that made it difficult to perform even the simplest tasks. He had lost weight, and his skin had a pallid, almost sallow look. It was clear that this was not a typical summer flu.

I conducted a thorough physical examination, noting his elevated temperature, rapid pulse, and labored breathing. His lungs sounded congested, and there was a noticeable rattle when he breathed. Given his worsening condition, I decided to run a series of blood tests and ordered a chest X-ray to rule out pneumonia or other respiratory infections.

The results were alarming. The chest X-ray showed significant inflammation in his lungs, but no clear signs of bacterial pneumonia. The blood tests revealed elevated white blood cell counts and liver enzymes, which suggested an infection but did not pinpoint a specific cause. His symptoms were severe, and the lack of a definitive diagnosis was concerning.

I consulted with a colleague, an infectious disease specialist, to review the patient's case. We discussed the possibility of a zoonotic infection, given his occupation and the rural environment he lived in. The specialist suggested testing for Q fever, a disease caused by the bacterium Coxiella burnetii. It was a long shot, but the symptoms fit, and the patient's occupation put him at risk.

The test for Q fever came back positive. Coxiellosis, as it is also known, is often contracted through inhalation of dust contaminated with the bacteria, which can come from the birth products, urine, feces, or milk of infected animals, particularly sheep, cattle, and goats. It was not a common diagnosis, but it explained the patient's array of symptoms and their severity.

With a diagnosis in hand, we began treatment immediately. The mainstay of therapy for acute Q fever is doxycycline, an antibiotic that is effective against the bacteria. I prescribed a two-week course of doxycycline and monitored the patient closely for any signs of improvement or adverse reactions to the medication.

In the initial days of treatment, there was little change in the patient's condition. He remained febrile, and his cough persisted. The headaches and muscle pains showed no sign of abating, and he became increasingly weak and fatigued. It was disheartening to see the lack of progress, but it was not entirely unexpected; Coxiellosis can be a stubborn infection.

As the first week of treatment drew to a close, there were the faintest signs of improvement. His fever began to subside, and he reported that his headaches were less severe. The cough, however, lingered, and his energy levels were still low. I encouraged him to maintain the course of antibiotics and assured him that it could take time for the full effects to be felt.

During the second week, his condition improved more noticeably. The fever resolved completely, and his cough became less frequent and productive. The muscle pains diminished, and he began to regain some of his lost weight. His appetite returned, and there was a bit of color in his cheeks once more. It seemed that the treatment was working.

However, Coxiellosis can have a chronic form, which can develop if the acute infection is not completely eradicated. This form can affect the heart, liver, and bones, leading to serious complications. Given the severity of his initial symptoms and the delayed response to treatment, I was concerned about the possibility of chronic Q fever.

I scheduled regular follow-ups to monitor his progress and conducted additional tests to check for any lingering signs of infection. The results were reassuring; his liver enzymes returned to normal, and there were no signs of endocarditis, a potentially life-threatening inflammation of the heart's inner lining that can occur with chronic Q fever.

Over the next few months, the patient's health continued to improve. He regained his strength and was able to return to his work on the farm. He remained under surveillance, with periodic blood tests to ensure that the infection had been fully eradicated. Each visit showed consistent improvements, and there were no signs of relapse.

Reflecting on his case, it was clear that an accurate and timely diagnosis was crucial to his recovery. Coxiellosis, though rare, can present with severe symptoms that mimic other illnesses, making it a challenging diagnosis. The patient's occupation and environment were key factors that pointed us in the right direction.

The experience also highlighted the importance of considering zoonotic diseases in patients with unexplained febrile illnesses, particularly those who are in frequent contact with animals. The patient's perseverance through the ordeal was commendable, and his eventual recovery was a testament to the effectiveness of the treatment when administered appropriately.

While he ultimately made a full recovery, his case served as a reminder of the complexities and potential severity of zoonotic infections. It underscored the need for vigilance and thorough investigation in patients with atypical presentations of common symptoms. Coxiellosis, though a rare diagnosis, was a significant learning experience that would undoubtedly influence my approach to future cases with similar presentations.

# CHAPTER NINETEEN

## DELLEMAN-OORTHUYS SYNDROME

THE PATIENT ARRIVED in my office one dreary November morning, carried by an air of desperation that clung to the autumn chill. The initial referral had been for an ophthalmological consultation due to frequent eye infections and discomfort, but a cursory glance at the patient revealed that there was more to the story. The asymmetry in their face was striking, an uneven terrain of swelling and depressions that piqued my curiosity. I noted the peculiar arrangement of hair follicles, with patches of alopecia interspersed with dense growths, like islands in a barren sea.

During the preliminary examination, the patient exhibited symptoms that resonated with an affliction I'd only encountered in medical journals: Delleman-Oorthuys syndrome, also known as oculocerebrocutaneous syndrome. This rare genetic disorder, with its triad of ocular, cerebral, and cutaneous anomalies, is as enigmatic as it is challenging to manage. I commenced a thorough assessment, beginning with the eyes, where the patient described recurrent infections and impaired vision. Examination revealed epibulbar dermoids, benign growths on the surface of the eye, and colobomas, congenital defects where normal tissue in or around the eye was absent.

Moving to the cutaneous anomalies, I observed linear skin defects, some of which were ulcerated and infected. These lesions, coupled with areas of hyperpigmentation and hypopigmentation, presented a complex dermatological challenge. The patient's scalp bore the hallmark of the syndrome: aplasia cutis congenita, areas where the skin had failed to develop properly, leaving patches of thin, fragile skin prone to tearing and infection.

The neurological evaluation was equally troubling. The patient had a history of seizures, and their cognitive abilities were below what would be expected for their age. Neuroimaging confirmed the presence of porencephalic cysts—fluid-filled cavities within the brain—and polymicrogyria, a condition characterized by abnormal brain development, leading to numerous small, misshapen gyri.

Diagnosing Delleman-Oorthuys syndrome was both a relief and a burden. It provided a name for the patient's suffering but also underscored the complexity of their condition. Treatment would not be straightforward, requiring a multidisciplinary approach to address the myriad symptoms. I began to formulate a plan, starting with the most pressing issues: the ocular and dermatological manifestations.

For the ocular problems, surgical intervention was necessary to remove the epibulbar dermoids and repair the colobomas as much as possible. The patient's frequent infections necessitated rigorous hygiene and prophylactic antibiotics to prevent further complications. Postoperative care included regular follow-ups to monitor healing and manage any emergent issues.

Dermatologically, the patient's lesions required meticulous care. We initiated a regimen of topical antibiotics and corticosteroids to manage the infections and inflammation. For the more severe ulcerations, surgical debridement was performed to remove necrotic tissue, followed by skin grafts to promote healing. The patient was also educated on wound care techniques to minimize the risk of future infections.

The neurological aspect of the treatment was perhaps the most daunting. The patient's seizures were poorly controlled, requiring a combination of antiepileptic drugs tailored to their specific needs. We also embarked on a rehabilitative program to address their cognitive impairments, involving speech therapy, occupational therapy, and special education services.

As the weeks turned into months, the patient's progress was incremental but noticeable. The ocular surgeries had significantly improved their vision, and the stringent hygiene practices reduced the frequency of infections. Dermatologically, the healing was slow but steady. The ulcerated lesions began to close, and the skin grafts took hold, providing a layer of protection against further damage. Neurologically, the seizure control was still a work in progress, with adjustments to medication dosages and types being a frequent necessity.

However, the journey was far from smooth. There were setbacks, particularly with the skin lesions, which would sometimes become reinfected despite our best efforts. Each new infection felt like a personal failure, a reminder of the relentless nature of the syndrome. The patient endured these challenges with a fortitude that was inspiring, their spirit unbroken despite the constant physical and emotional toll.

The patient's support system, consisting of family and a network of caregivers, played a crucial role in their care. Their dedication was evident in the way they adhered to the treatment protocols, provided comfort during the frequent hospital visits, and maintained a positive environment for the patient. This collective effort was instrumental in the gradual improvements we witnessed.

As we moved into the second year of treatment, there were moments of hope interspersed with periods of despair. The patient's vision had stabilized, and they reported a significant reduction in discomfort. The skin lesions, although still present, were less severe and more manageable. Neurologically, the seizure frequency had decreased, and the patient showed modest improvements in cognitive functions, thanks to the relentless efforts of the therapy team.

Yet, despite these gains, the underlying condition remained a formidable adversary. The patient's immune system was compromised, making them susceptible to infections that could quickly escalate. Each hospital admission for an infection brought a cascade of complications, from antibiotic resistance to the emotional strain on the patient and their family.

One particularly harsh winter, the patient was admitted with a severe respiratory infection. This time, the battle proved too much for their weakened body. Despite aggressive treatment, including intravenous antibiotics, respiratory support, and intensive care, the infection spread, leading to sepsis. The patient's organs began to fail, one by one, despite our best efforts to stabilize them.

In those final days, the intensive care unit became a somber place. The constant beeping of monitors, the sterile scent of antiseptics, and the hushed conversations of medical staff created an atmosphere of quiet desperation. The patient's family remained by their side, their faces etched with sorrow and fatigue. We tried everything within our power, but the combination of Delleman-Oorthuys syndrome and the severe infection was insurmountable.

When the end came, it was peaceful. The patient slipped away, surrounded by loved ones, their suffering finally at an end. The quiet that followed was heavy with grief but also with a sense of release. The relentless struggle against a cruel and unyielding condition had ceased.

In the aftermath, as I reviewed the patient's journey, I was struck by the sheer complexity and the multifaceted nature of their condition. Delleman-Oorthuys syndrome had presented a unique set of challenges, pushing the boundaries of my medical knowledge and emotional endurance. Each aspect of the syndrome required a different approach, a different kind of expertise, and a collective effort that spanned multiple disciplines.

In the end, the patient's journey with Delleman-Oorthuys syndrome was a mosaic of pain and perseverance, of fleeting victories and profound losses. Their life, though marked by suffering, also revealed the depths of compassion and dedication that define the practice of medicine.

# CHAPTER TWENTY

## MADELUNG'S DISEASE

I HAD BEEN a physician for nearly two decades when I first encountered Madelung's disease, also known as multiple symmetric lipomatosis. The patient, a middle-aged individual, came to me with a perplexing array of symptoms. Their appearance was the first thing that struck me – the neck was notably thickened, as were the upper arms and upper back. These areas were not merely swollen; they had a distinct, soft, rubbery texture that suggested an unusual form of adipose tissue accumulation.

Initially, the patient's complaints were vague: fatigue, discomfort, and difficulty with physical activities that they previously managed with ease. The discomfort was not sharp or acute but rather a persistent, dull ache that seemed to be exacerbated by movement and certain positions. I conducted a thorough physical examination, noting the symmetrical deposits of fat that seemed to encircle the neck like a grotesque collar. This was not typical obesity; the distribution was too localized and peculiar.

Suspecting a metabolic or endocrine disorder, I ordered a series of tests. Blood work revealed normal lipid levels and thyroid function, which ruled out more common conditions like hypothyroidism or hyperlipidemia. Given the unusual presentation and my growing suspicion, I decided to delve into less common disorders. After consulting medical literature and discussing with a colleague who specialized in rare diseases, I considered Madelung's disease a likely diagnosis.

To confirm, I ordered imaging studies. An MRI provided the clearest picture – extensive lipomatous deposits in the cervico-thoracic region, sparing other areas typically involved in obesity. This imaging, combined with the clinical presentation, confirmed the diagnosis of Madelung's disease. The patient exhibited classic features: symmetrical, painless fatty masses predominantly in the upper body, with no significant metabolic abnormalities.

Breaking the news to the patient was challenging. Madelung's disease is rare and largely idiopathic, meaning its exact cause is unknown, though it has been associated with chronic alcoholism and mitochondrial dysfunction. The patient had no history of alcohol abuse, which made the etiology even more perplexing. I explained that the condition is progressive and currently has no definitive cure, but various management strategies could alleviate symptoms and potentially slow progression.

The initial management focused on symptomatic relief and monitoring. We discussed lifestyle modifications, including diet and exercise, although these would have limited impact on the lipomatous deposits themselves. I referred the patient to a nutritionist to ensure they were receiving balanced meals, avoiding potential metabolic triggers.

Pain management became a priority. Although the patient's discomfort was not debilitating, it significantly impacted their quality of life. I prescribed nonsteroidal anti-inflammatory drugs (NSAIDs) to address the pain and inflammation. Additionally, I suggested physical therapy to maintain mobility and prevent muscle atrophy due to decreased physical activity. The physical therapist worked with the patient to design a regimen that accommodated their limitations while promoting overall strength and flexibility.

Despite these efforts, the disease's progression was relentless. Over the following months, the fatty masses increased in size, further restricting the patient's range of motion and exacerbating their discomfort. The weight of the deposits on the neck and shoulders began to affect their posture, causing chronic neck and back pain. I consulted with a surgical colleague to explore the possibility of liposuction or surgical excision of the fatty masses. While surgery could provide temporary relief, it was not a definitive solution and carried risks, including infection, scarring, and recurrence of the lipomas.

After careful consideration, the patient opted for surgical intervention. The procedure aimed to remove the most burdensome masses to improve mobility and reduce pain. The surgery was technically challenging due to the extensive vascular supply to the lipomas and their proximity to vital structures. Nonetheless, it was successful, and the patient experienced significant relief post-operatively. The neck and upper arms appeared more natural, and their range of motion improved noticeably.

However, the respite was short-lived. Within a year, the lipomas began to recur, as anticipated. The patient's frustration was palpable, and I felt a deep empathy for their plight. We continued with conservative management, integrating new pain relief techniques such as nerve blocks and exploring alternative therapies like acupuncture. Psychological support was also crucial; the chronic nature of the disease and its impact on appearance and function took a toll on the patient's mental health. I referred them to a counselor experienced in dealing with chronic illness to provide emotional support and coping strategies.

As the disease advanced, complications arose. The increasing size of the lipomas around the neck began to compress the airway, causing sleep apnea and respiratory difficulties. This was a grave development, necessitating the involvement of a pulmonologist. The patient was fitted with a continuous positive airway pressure (CPAP) device to assist with breathing during sleep. Despite these measures, their condition continued to deteriorate.

Nutritional status became another concern. The bulkiness of the lipomas around the neck made swallowing difficult, leading to weight loss and malnutrition. I collaborated with a dietitian to devise a high-calorie, easily digestible diet to ensure the patient received adequate nutrition without exacerbating their discomfort. We considered enteral feeding as a last resort, but the patient was determined to maintain oral intake as long as possible.

Over time, the patient's ability to perform daily activities diminished. Simple tasks like dressing, bathing, and eating became arduous, requiring assistance. I coordinated with a home health care team to provide the necessary support. This included occupational therapy to adapt the patient's living environment and maximize their independence. The therapists introduced adaptive devices and techniques to facilitate self-care and mobility, striving to preserve the patient's dignity and quality of life.

Despite our best efforts, the disease's inexorable progression led to severe disability. The patient became increasingly dependent on others for basic needs, a situation they found deeply demoralizing. They expressed feelings of isolation and despair, grappling with the reality of a condition that had no cure and little hope for improvement.

In the final stages of the disease, the patient developed respiratory failure due to the extensive lipomatous deposits compressing the airway and lungs. This marked a critical turning point. We initiated palliative care to focus on comfort and quality of life rather than curative measures. The goal was to alleviate pain and distress, ensuring the patient's remaining time was as comfortable as possible.

The end came quietly. Surrounded by loved ones and under the compassionate care of the palliative team, the patient passed away peacefully. Their journey through Madelung's disease had been fraught with challenges, pain, and relentless progression. As a physician, I was left with a profound sense of sorrow and reflection. This case highlighted the limitations of medical science in the face of rare and incurable diseases, underscoring the importance of compassion, comprehensive care, and the human element in medicine.

The experience profoundly impacted my approach to patient care. It reinforced the necessity of empathy, patient-centered care, and the need for ongoing research into rare diseases. Madelung's disease remains a challenging condition with no definitive treatment, but each patient's story contributes to the broader understanding and potential future breakthroughs. Through this patient's journey, I was reminded of the resilience of the human spirit and the vital role of a supportive medical team in navigating the complexities of chronic illness.

Continue with
Crazy Medical Stories: Volume 2

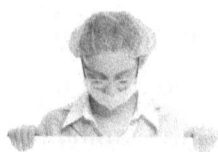

CRAZY MEDICAL STORIES

VOLUME 2

DR. ERIN SMITH

## ABOUT THE AUTHOR

Dr. Erin Smith is a distinguished physician and author, originally hailing from the warm, vibrant landscapes of Alabama. With a career spanning over two decades, she has carved a niche for herself in the medical field, earning respect and admiration from colleagues and patients alike. Dr. Smith's journey in medicine has been marked by her unwavering dedication, sharp intellect, and a heartfelt passion for making a difference in the lives of others.

After completing her medical training in Alabama, Dr. Smith decided to spread her wings and bring her Southern charm and expertise to new horizons. She eventually settled outside of Salt Lake City, where she has continued to thrive both professionally and personally.

In addition to her demanding career, Dr. Smith is a devoted wife and the proud mother of two energetic sons. Balancing her professional responsibilities with her role as a mother has been a rewarding challenge, and she credits her family for providing her with the strength and support to excel in every facet of her life.

Dr. Smith's unique ability to connect with her patients, combined with her flair for storytelling, led her to compile and share her wealth of experiences in her book, *Crazy Medical Stories*. In this anthology, she opens up a window to the fascinating world of medicine, showcasing the unpredictable, the miraculous, and the bizarre stories she has encountered over her illustrious career.

With her roots firmly planted in her Alabama heritage, and her branches extending to nurture her family and career in Utah, Dr. Erin Smith stands as a remarkable figure in medicine—a doctor with a heart as big as her intellect, and stories as captivating as her journey.

ALSO BY FREE REIGN PUBLISHING

LEGENDS AND STORIES: FROM THE
APPALACHIAN TRAIL

10-33: TRUE TALES FROM THE THIN BLUE LINE

TERROR IN THE WOODS

www.ingramcontent.com/pod-product-compliance
Lightning Source LLC
Chambersburg PA
CBHW022040190326
41520CB00008B/663